NATIONAL ACADEMIES
Sciences
Engineering
Medicine

NATIONAL ACADEMIES PRESS
Washington, DC

Improving the CDC Quarantine Station Network's Response to Emerging Threats

Committee on the Analysis to Enhance the Effectiveness of the Federal Quarantine Station Network based on Lessons from the COVID-19 Pandemic

Board on Global Health

Board on Population Health and Public Health Practice

Health and Medicine Division

Consensus Study Report

THE NATIONAL ACADEMIES PRESS 500 Fifth Street, NW Washington, DC 20001

This activity was supported by contracts between the National Academy of Sciences and U.S. Centers for Disease Control and Prevention (75D30121F0010). Any opinions, findings, conclusions, or recommendations expressed in this publication do not necessarily reflect the views of any organization or agency that provided support for the project.

International Standard Book Number-13: 978-0-309-68969-4
International Standard Book Number-10: 0-309-68969-4
Digital Object Identifier: https://doi.org/10.17226/26599
Library of Congress Catalog Number: 2022943211

This publication is available from the National Academies Press, 500 Fifth Street, NW, Keck 360, Washington, DC 20001; (800) 624-6242 or (202) 334-3313; http://www.nap.edu.

Copyright 2022 by the National Academy of Sciences. National Academies of Sciences, Engineering, and Medicine and National Academies Press and the graphical logos for each are all trademarks of the National Academy of Sciences. All rights reserved.

Printed in the United States of America

Suggested citation: National Academies of Sciences, Engineering, and Medicine. 2022. *Improving the CDC Quarantine Station Network's response to emerging threats*. Washington, DC: The National Academies Press. https://doi.org/10.17226/26599.

The **National Academy of Sciences** was established in 1863 by an Act of Congress, signed by President Lincoln, as a private, nongovernmental institution to advise the nation on issues related to science and technology. Members are elected by their peers for outstanding contributions to research. Dr. Marcia McNutt is president.

The **National Academy of Engineering** was established in 1964 under the charter of the National Academy of Sciences to bring the practices of engineering to advising the nation. Members are elected by their peers for extraordinary contributions to engineering. Dr. John L. Anderson is president.

The **National Academy of Medicine** (formerly the Institute of Medicine) was established in 1970 under the charter of the National Academy of Sciences to advise the nation on medical and health issues. Members are elected by their peers for distinguished contributions to medicine and health. Dr. Victor J. Dzau is president.

The three Academies work together as the **National Academies of Sciences, Engineering, and Medicine** to provide independent, objective analysis and advice to the nation and conduct other activities to solve complex problems and inform public policy decisions. The National Academies also encourage education and research, recognize outstanding contributions to knowledge, and increase public understanding in matters of science, engineering, and medicine.

Learn more about the National Academies of Sciences, Engineering, and Medicine at **www.nationalacademies.org**.

Consensus Study Reports published by the National Academies of Sciences, Engineering, and Medicine document the evidence-based consensus on the study's statement of task by an authoring committee of experts. Reports typically include findings, conclusions, and recommendations based on information gathered by the committee and the committee's deliberations. Each report has been subjected to a rigorous and independent peer-review process and it represents the position of the National Academies on the statement of task.

Proceedings published by the National Academies of Sciences, Engineering, and Medicine chronicle the presentations and discussions at a workshop, symposium, or other event convened by the National Academies. The statements and opinions contained in proceedings are those of the participants and are not endorsed by other participants, the planning committee, or the National Academies.

Rapid Expert Consultations published by the National Academies of Sciences, Engineering, and Medicine are authored by subject-matter experts on narrowly focused topics that can be supported by a body of evidence. The discussions contained in rapid expert consultations are considered those of the authors and do not contain policy recommendations. Rapid expert consultations are reviewed by the institution before release.

For information about other products and activities of the National Academies, please visit www.nationalacademies.org/about/whatwedo.

COMMITTEE ON THE ANALYSIS TO ENHANCE THE EFFECTIVENESS OF THE FEDERAL QUARANTINE STATION NETWORK BASED ON LESSONS FROM THE COVID-19 PANDEMIC

GEORGES C. BENJAMIN (*Chair*), Executive Director, American Public Health Association
ANA ABRAÍDO-LANZA, Vice Dean and Professor, Department of Social and Behavioral Sciences, School of Global Public Health, New York University
MICHELE BARRY, Drs. Ben and A. Jess Shenson Professor of Medicine and Tropical Diseases and Senior Associate Dean for Global Health, Stanford University
IETZA BOJORQUEZ, Professor, Department of Population Studies, El Colegio de la Frontera Norte, Mexico
BRADLEY DICKERSON, Senior Manager, Chemical and Biological Security, Sandia National Laboratories
LAWRENCE O. GOSTIN, Founding Linda D. & Timothy J. O'Neill Professor of Global Health Law; and Director, WHO Collaborating Center on National and Global Health Law
MOON KIM, Medical Epidemiologist, Los Angeles County Department of Public Health Acute Communicable Disease Control Program
LONNIE KING, Academy Professor and Dean Emeritus, College of Veterinary Medicine, The Ohio State University
MARCELLE LAYTON, Chief Medical Officer, Council of State and Territorial Epidemiologists
STEPHEN OSTROFF, Adjunct Professor, University of Pittsburgh Graduate School of Public Health
EDWARD T. RYAN, Director of Global Infectious Diseases, Massachusetts General Hospital; Professor, Harvard University
ALESSANDRO VESPIGNANI, Sternberg Family Distinguished Professor and Director, Network Science Institute, Northeastern University
C. JASON WANG, Professor of Pediatrics and Health Policy, Stanford University
RUEBEN WARREN, Professor of Bioethics and Director of the National Center for Bioethics in Research and Health Care, Tuskegee University

Study Staff

TEQUAM WORKU, Study Director
ELIZABETH ASHBY, Associate Program Officer

ELIZABETH FERRÉ, Research Associate
EMILIE RYAN-CASTILLO, Research Assistant
JULIE PAVLIN, Senior Director, Board on Global Health
ROSE MARIE MARTINEZ, Senior Director, Board on Population Health and Public Health Practice

Consultants

NIXON ARAUZ, Mirzayan Fellow, Virginia Commonwealth University
BENJAMIN BURK, American University, School of Public Affairs
GENIE GROHMAN, Editor
TAMARA HAAG, Science Writer
WASAN KUMAR, Stanford University School of Medicine
ANNA NICHOLSON, Science Writer
LINDSAY WILEY, UCLA School of Law

Reviewers

This Consensus Study Report was reviewed in draft form by individuals chosen for their diverse perspectives and technical expertise. The purpose of this independent review is to provide candid and critical comments that will assist the National Academies of Sciences, Engineering, and Medicine in making each published report as sound as possible and to ensure that it meets the institutional standards for quality, objectivity, evidence, and responsiveness to the study charge. The review comments and draft manuscript remain confidential to protect the integrity of the deliberative process.

We thank the following individuals for their review of this report:

R. ALTA CHARO, J.D., University of Wisconsin
CARLOS DEL RIO, M.D., Emory University
SIMON I. HAY, DPhil, DSc, FMedSci, University of Washington
JAMES G. HODGE, JR., J.D., LLM, Arizona State University
ERIC MCDONALD, M.D., M.P.H., FACEP, County of San Diego, Health and Human Services Agency
MARCUS PLESCIA, M.D., M.P.H., Association of State and Territorial Health Officials (ASTHO)
JAY J. SCHNITZER, M.D., Ph.D., The MITRE Corporation
JAIME SEPULVEDA, M.D., DSc, M.P.H., University of California, San Francisco

Although the reviewers listed above provided many constructive comments and suggestions, they were not asked to endorse the conclusions or recommendations of this report nor did they see the final draft before its release. The review of this report was overseen by **MARLA SALMON,** University of Washington, and **TERRY McELWAIN,** Washington State University.

They were responsible for making certain that an independent examination of this report was carried out in accordance with the standards of the National Academies and that all review comments were carefully considered. Responsibility for the final content rests entirely with the authoring committee and the National Academies.

Acknowledgments

This report would not be possible without the sponsorship of the Centers for Disease Control and Prevention Division of Global Migration and Quarantine, whose affiliates were instrumental in conceptualizing the study's statement of task. The committee wishes to extend its immense gratitude to the many experts who lent their time to presentations during public sessions and who provided invaluable insights to the study. Their names and affiliations can be found in the committee meeting agendas in Appendix B.

The National Academies staff wish to acknowledge Tina Seliber, Leslie Sim, and Taryn Young, for their coordination during the review process, as well as to Lauren Shern for providing guidance throughout the course of the project. The staff also thank Victor Stewart for managing the contract throughout the life cycle of the study. The staff also extend their gratitude to Chloe O'Connor from the Research Center for her assistance with fact checking.

Preface

The concept of quarantine has been around since the 14th century. When used appropriately, it has been a proven strategy for mitigating the impact of various contagious diseases. Back then, the quarantine process primarily consisted of holding an arriving ship at sea for 40 days to prevent nearby communities from contracting the plague or another infectious disease. This concept has survived through the ages and in 1878 the U.S. Congress passed the first federal quarantine law. Over the years, the federal government became more concerned about infectious disease control at our borders and between states. In 1944 it passed the Public Health Service Act, which modernized the U.S. Public Health Service and with it enhanced its ability to address disease control including infectious diseases. It also gave it the prime responsibility for controlling onward transmission of communicable diseases.

The U.S. Centers for Disease Control and Prevention (CDC) now has oversight for preventing the entry, transmission, and spread of communicable diseases of public health concern into the United States from other nations. It does this primarily through its Division of Global Migration and Quarantine (DGMQ). This division has undergone major changes through the years, both on the scope of its responsibility and its approach to disease control. In 2004 the DGMQ asked the Institute of Medicine of the National Academies of Sciences, Engineering, and Medicine (the National Academies) to assess the present CDC quarantine stations and recommend how they should evolve to meet the challenges posed by microbial threats at the nation's gateways. The DGMQ specifically requested "an assessment of the role of the federal quarantine stations, given the changes in the global environment including large increases in international travel, threats posed by bioterrorism and emerging infections, and the movement of animals and cargo."

The Institute of Medicine (IOM) committee charged with the assessment did a comprehensive review and made several recommendations in its 2006 report titled *Quarantine Stations at Ports of Entry: Protecting the Public's Health* which the DGMQ believes helped it guide and improve its functions and prepare for the future. In many ways, the DGMQ believes the federal quarantine station network has improved its service delivery as well as the scientific basis of its decision making in addressing the disease threats the country has experienced in recent years.

The 2006 report came in the aftermath of the severe acute respiratory syndrome (SARS) epidemic of 2003–2004.[1] Since then, the world has experienced multiple public health emergencies of international concern, including from the Zika and Ebola viruses and H1N1 influenza (influenza A virus subtype H1N1, also known as swine flu). In December 2019 a novel coronavirus outbreak began in Wuhan, China, and has become the worst pandemic of a respiratory virus since the influenza pandemic of 1918. Known as the COVID-19 pandemic, it is caused by a newly evolved coronavirus—SARS-CoV-2. The COVID-19 pandemic, which as of this writing is ongoing, has had a profound impact throughout the world and has challenged the public health systems of every country. It has also led to a reevaluation of many of our current disease control mechanisms, including the use and role of quarantine as a public health tool.

The COVID pandemic, as of May 23, 2022, has caused over 520,000,000 reported cases worldwide and over 6,200,000 reported deaths, including over 83,345,820 documented cases and 1,002,283 deaths in the United States alone. However, these figures are a great underestimate of the true burden. The quarantine system of the United States has been tested like never before. The use of isolation and quarantine authority during the COVID-19 pandemic in the United States has included international border closures, limits to transportation, and even suspension of the cruise industry. Physical distancing recommendations by public health authorities resulted in wide-scale implementation of isolation and quarantine practices. Emerging technologies for the identification of febrile individuals and the tracking of potentially exposed or infected individuals, using cellular phones and COVID-19 testing as a requirement for international travelers, were used as a component of the quarantine function in various nations. The science and evidence for the effectiveness of these measures remains under study today. As of this writing, the COVID-19 pandemic appears to

---

[1] This text was modified after release of the report to the study sponsor to correct the dates of SARS epidemic.

be slowly transitioning to another phase, possibly an endemic phase. The DGMQ must not only continue its current activities, but must also learn from the federal quarantine station network's response to the pandemic in order to evolve and be better prepared to provide the strategic leadership and operations necessary to protect the nation.

Because of the need to be forward leaning for significant threats like COVID-19 in the future, in 2021, the DGMQ has again asked the National Academies to evaluate the effectiveness of the Federal Quarantine Station Network based on lessons from the COVID-19 pandemic. Once again, a committee of the Academies looked at the operating environment, organizational structure, and legal framework; the workforce and its culture; functional relationships and partnerships; and supporting resources. This assessment was informed by the domestic and international response to COVID-19 and by what is known to date about the successes and failures of the U.S. Federal Quarantine Network and other international disease control efforts. This pandemic is rapidly moving with a pathogen that is ever evolving. With that understanding, the committee focused on strategic and systemic issues and partnerships that we believe will survive the test of time, and strengthen the DGMQ network for the future.

This report was further informed by a committee of expert practitioners who brought their experience and knowledge base to ask probing questions and seek a better understanding of the information presented to us that informed our analysis. I also want to recognize the National Academies' dedicated professional staff, whose advice, expert background research, and gentle guidance was essential and without whom evidence-based reports of this type could not be produced.

Georges C. Benjamin, M.D., *Chair*
Committee on Analysis to Enhance the Effectiveness
of the Federal Quarantine Station Network Based
on Lessons Learned from the COVID-19 Pandemic

Contents

ACRONYMS AND ABBREVIATIONS   xix

SUMMARY   1

1   INTRODUCTION   17
    Charge to the Committee, 18
    Current Federal Quarantine Station Network, 21
    2006 IOM Report and Subsequent Developments, 25
    Structure of the Report, 27
    References, 28

2   ORGANIZATIONAL CAPACITY   31
    DGMQ Infrastructure, 32
    DGMQ'S Financial Landscape, 41
    Workforce, 46
    Culture, 59
    Conclusions and Recommendations, 60
    References, 65

3   DISEASE CONTROL AND RESPONSE EFFORTS   69
    The DGMQ's Roles and Responsibilities in Communicable
        Disease Control, 69
    Improving Strategic Planning for Potential Disease Outbreaks, 86
    Border Measures and Active Monitoring of International
        Travelers during COVID-19: Evaluation, 90

Conclusions and Recommendations, 97
References, 100

4 NEW TECHNOLOGIES AND DATA SYSTEMS   **107**
COVID-19 Detection Technologies, 108
Use of Innovative and Integrative Digital Technologies, 109
Leveraging Novel Digital Data Streams to Improve Situational Awareness, 118
Interoperability of Data Systems, 123
Balancing Ethical Risks with Public Health Benefits, 131
Conclusions and Recommendations, 139
References, 141

5 IMPROVING COORDINATION AND COLLABORATION   **149**
Collaboration with Key Partners, 150
Best Practices for Improving Coordination and Collaboration, 160
Elements of Effective Coordination and Collaboration, 162
Conclusions and Recommendations, 165
References, 168

6 LEGAL AND REGULATORY AUTHORITY   **171**
The CDC's Legal and Regulatory Authority during Outbreaks: Overview, 172
Recent Court Interpretations of the CDC's Authority, 173
Modernizing the CDC's Pandemic Prevention and Response Authority, 190
Surge Funding for Outbreak Response, 197
Conclusions and Recommendations, 202
References, 204

APPENDIXES
A BIOGRAPHICAL SKETCHES OF COMMITTEE MEMBERS AND STAFF   **207**
B AGENDAS: OPEN COMMITTEE MEETINGS   **217**

Boxes, Figures, and Tables

BOXES

1-1   Statement of Task, 19
1-2   Roles and Responsibilities of DGMQ Quarantine Stations, 24

3-1   Responsibilities of the Immigrant, Refugee, and Migrant Health (IRMH) Branch, 79
3-2   The DGMQ Emergency Response Activities during the COVID-19 Pandemic, 87
3-3   The CDC Center for Forecasting and Outbreak Analytics, 97

4-1   Connectathons of the Integrating the Healthcare Enterprise, 130

6-1   Proposed Quarantining of Diamond Cruise Ship Passengers, 183

FIGURES

1-1   CDC quarantine stations and their jurisdictions, 22

2-1   Organizational chart, Quarantine and Border Health Services Branch (QBHSB), 35
2-2   DGMQ's 10-year budget trends, 42
2-3   Quarantine and Border Health Services Branch (QBHSB) total staffing, 2008–2022, 49

xvii

2-4   Focus areas for DGMQ culture, 60

5-1   Federal governmental regulatory agencies for animal importation at ports of entry, 151

5-2   Complementary missions of the Department of Homeland Security and the Division of Global Migration and Quarantine, 153

TABLES

3-1   Potential Prioritization Scheme for Categorization of Pathogens, 88

4-1   Proximity and Location Awareness Technologies Used in Digital Contact Tracing and Tracking, 112

5-1   Recommendations from Council of State and Territorial Epidemiologists to CDC on Outbreak Response, 161

6-1   Powers Granted to the CDC by the Public Health Service Act of 1944, 175

6-2   Orders Issued by the DGMQ since COVID-19, 180

Acronyms and Abbreviations

ACF	Administration for Children and Families
ACIP	Advisory Committee on Immunization Practices
AIMS	Association of Public Health Laboratories Informatics Messaging Services
APA	Administrative Procedure Act
APHIS	Animal and Plant Health Inspection Service
APHL	Association of Public Health Laboratories
API	application programming interfaces
APIS	Advance Passenger Information System
ASPR	Office of the Assistant Secretary for Preparedness and Response
ASTHO	Association of State and Territorial Health Officials
ATS	Automated Targeting System
BIDS	Binational Infectious Disease Surveillance
BLE	Bluetooth Low Energy
CBP	U.S. Customs and Border Protection
CBRN	Chemical, Biological, Radiological and Nuclear Office
C-CDA	consolidated-clinical document architecture
CDC	U.S. Centers for Disease Control and Prevention
CDRP	communicable disease response plan
CEHR	certified electronic health record
CMS	Centers for Medicare & Medicaid Services
ComET	Communication, Evaluation, and Training, HHS

COOPERA	COVID-19: Operation for Personalized Empowerment to Render smart prevention And care seeking
COVID-19	Coronavirus Disease of 2019
CRA	Congressional Review Act
CSTE	Council of State and Territorial Epidemiologists
CWMD	Countering Weapons of Mass Destruction Office
DGMQ	Division of Global Migration and Quarantine, HHS
DHS	U.S. Department of Homeland Security
DNB	do not board
DoD	U.S. Department of Defense
DOI	U.S. Department of the Interior
DOJ	U.S. Department of Justice
DOS	U.S. Department of State
DOT	U.S. Department of Transportation
DP-3T	Decentralized Privacy-Preserving Proximity Tracing
DRF	Disaster Relief Fund
DSAT	Division of Select Agents and Toxins
Ebola	Ebola virus disease
ECG	electrocardiography
eCR	electronic case reporting
EDC	Enhanced Data Collection
eFIT	Epidemiology Field Team, HHS
EHR	electronic health record
EIOS	Epidemic Intelligence from Open Sources
ELR	electronic laboratory reporting
ENACT	Encounter-Based Architecture for Contact Tracing
EOC	CDC Emergency Operations Center
FAA	Federal Aviation Administration
FDA	U.S. Food and Drug Administration
FEMA	U.S. Federal Emergency Management Agency
FHIR	Fast Healthcare Interoperability Resources
FLETC	Federal Law Enforcement Training Center
FTE	full-time equivalent
FWS	U.S. Fish and Wildlife Services
FY	fiscal year
GAO	U.S. Government Accountability Office
GIS	geographic information system
GNSS	global navigation satellite system
GOARN	WHO's Global Outbreak Alert and Response Network

GPHIN	Global Public Health Intelligence Network
GPS	global positioning system
GS	general schedule
H1N1	Influenza A virus subtype H1N1, aka swine flu
HHS	U.S. Department of Health and Human Services
HIN	health information network
HIPAA	The Health Insurance Portability and Accountability Act
HR	human resources
ICE	Immigration and Customs Enforcement
IHE	Integrating the Healthcare Enterprise
IHR	International Health Regulations
IRMH	Immigrant, Refugee, and Migrant Health branch
JHU CSSE	Johns Hopkins University's Center for Systems Science and Engineering
LAMP	loop-mediated isothermal amplification
MDR-TB	Multidrug-resistant tuberculosis
MERS	Middle Eastern Respiratory Syndrome
mNGS	Metagenomics Next-generation Sequencing
MOA	Memorandum of Agreement
MOU	Memorandum of Understanding
NACCHO	The National Association of County and City Health Officials
NCEZID	National Center for Emerging and Zoonotic Infectious Disease
NFC	near-field communication
NHS	National Health Service
NPI	nonpharmaceutical intervention
OAW	Operation Allies Welcome
OC	organizational capacity
OGA	Office of Global Affairs
OMB	Office of Management and Budget, HHS
ONC	Office of the National Coordinator for Health Information Technology
ORR	Office of Refugee Resettlement
PCR	polymerase chain reaction

PDPH	Philadelphia Department of Public Health
PHE	public health emergency
PHEF	The Public Health Emergency Fund
PHSA	Public Health Service Act of 1944
PKEMRA	Post-Katrina Emergency Response Act
PNR	Passenger Name Record
POE	port of entry or point of entry
PPCT	Preparedness and Policy Coordination Team, HHS
PPE	personal protective equipment
ProMED	International Society for Infectious Diseases' Program for Monitoring Emerging Diseases
QARS	Quarantine Activity Reporting System
QBHSB	Quarantine and Boarder Health Services Branch, HHS
QR	Quick Response
QuarTET	Quarantine Travel Epidemiology Team, HHS
RFID	radio-frequency identification
RSST	Resource Support Services Team
RT-PCR	reverse transcription polymerase chain reaction
SARS-CoV-1	severe acute respiratory syndrome coronavirus 1
SARS-CoV-2	severe acute respiratory syndrome coronavirus 2
SNS	Strategic National Stockpile
SOP	standard operating procedure
STLT	state, tribal, local, and territorial
TB	tuberculosis
TEFCA	Trusted Exchange Framework and Common Agreement
TERM NTE	temporary federal appointee
TSA	Transportation Security Administration
UCG	Unified Coordination Group
USAID	U.S. Agency for International Development
USCG	U.S. Coast Guard
USDA	U.S. Department of Agriculture
USG	U.S. government
USMU	The United States–Mexico Health Unit
USSD	unstructured supplementary service data
VHD	Virginia Health Department
VSP	Vessel Sanitation Program

WHO	World Health Organization
XDR-TB	extensively drug-resistant tuberculosis
ZTeam	Zoonoses Team, HHS, CDC

Summary

The federal network of quarantine stations spans ports of entry across the United States, serving as a premier line of defense against the importation of infectious disease threats across the nation's borders through travelers arriving by air, land, and sea. The United States typically receives nearly 1 million travelers per day into the country, underscoring the need for a rapid, nimble, and effective response when travelers with communicable diseases of public health concern are identified. To help prevent the introduction, transmission, and spread of communicable diseases across and within the country, the Division of Global Migration and Quarantine (DGMQ) within the Centers for Disease Control and Prevention (CDC) operates quarantine stations staffed by public health officers at 20 U.S. international airports and land-border crossings with the highest concentrations of incoming international travelers.

Over the past two decades, the public health, social, and economic threats posed by infectious diseases—particularly due to emerging pathogens of epidemic and pandemic potential—have intensified significantly, compounded by the increasing ease, speed, and range of international travel. Consequently, the DGMQ has faced an increasing number of emergency public health responses during that period, most recently COVID-19. Estimates show that more than 3.4 billion people worldwide may have been infected with SARS-CoV-2 (Barber et al., 2022). Excess mortality resulting from the pandemic could be over 18 million (Wang et al., 2022), highlighting the devastating consequences of limited capacities to mitigate and control the introduction, transmission, and spread of emerging and reemerging infectious pathogens such as novel coronaviruses. Beyond the ongoing COVID-19 pandemic, the world in recent years has had to respond to SARS, MERS (Middle East respiratory syndrome), Zika, West Nile Virus, and multiple Ebola virus disease epidemics and outbreaks.

In 2004, catalyzed by concerns about bioterrorism and emerging infectious disease threats, the CDC requested that the Institute of Medicine (IOM) conduct a consensus study to recommend strategies to strengthen the DGMQ's quarantine station network, resulting in the report *Quarantine Stations at Ports of Entry: Protecting the Public's Health* (Institute of Medicine, 2006). Similarly, in 2021, the CDC called upon the National Academies of Sciences, Engineering, and Medicine (the National Academies) to conduct another evaluation of the DGMQ's role and the federal quarantine station network in mitigating the risk of onward transmission of microbial threats by drawing upon lessons learned from the response to the COVID-19 pandemic and other recent emergency responses. The National Academies appointed an ad hoc committee of experts to fulfill this request. Specifically, the committee was charged with assessing the role of DGMQ quarantine stations in mitigating the risk of onward communicable disease transmission in light of changes in the global environment, including large increases in international travel, threats posed by emerging infections, and the movement of animals and cargo.

The landscape has changed substantially since the IOM report in 2006, not only in terms of the increasing emergence of novel pathogens and burgeoning international travel, but also in terms of the number of quarantine stations, increases in DGMQ's responsibilities without commensurate increases in baseline funding and personnel, changes in the legal landscape for emergency responses and national security protections, evolving roles of the World Health Organization (WHO) and other transnational entities, and the advent of a host of new technologies and data sources that could be leveraged to support disease control.

The committee acknowledges that the DGMQ has implemented many successful changes and activities since the earlier report. Yet, extraordinary infectious disease events have occurred in the last 15 years along with their significant impacts on the DGMQ. The findings and recommendations of this report are not a reflection of any failure by the DGMQ and its outstanding staff, but, rather, a reflection of the difficult times and circumstances in which the division has had to work to try to achieve its valuable mission.

The committee's findings and recommendations span five domains: (1) opportunities to strengthen the DGMQ's organizational capacity, including its infrastructure; (2) strategies to mitigate the risk of importing infectious threats into the country and to improve response efforts; (3) methods to optimize the use of novel technologies and data systems to detect and track infectious threats; (4) approaches to improve coordination and collaboration to enhance disease control; and (5) ways to modernize the CDC legal and regulatory authority to more effectively respond to public health threats.

ORGANIZATIONAL CAPACITY

Organizational capacity (OC) refers to an institution's ability to perform critical tasks and fulfill its mission. As the entity responsible for disease surveillance at U.S. ports of entry, the DGMQ's OC is a critical element of U.S. national health security. The committee identified and evaluated the four key areas that directly influence the DGMQ's ability to complete its core tasks: infrastructure, finances, workforce, and organizational culture.

The DGMQ's infrastructure is central to its OC and is a key element in protecting public health as people become increasingly mobile within today's globally interconnected world. One branch within the DGMQ, the Quarantine and Border Health Services Branch (QBHSB), holds primary responsibility for both monitoring incoming travelers for diseases of public health concern and planning for emergency response. All but two of the twenty quarantine stations are under the jurisdiction of the QBHSB. The committee noted that the DGMQ has a unique set of responsibilities and is one of the few units at the CDC with direct regulatory responsibilities. It is also one of the few CDC divisions that has a network of operational field units, including those with international responsibilities.

Finances are foundational to the other critical elements of OC. Despite the increasing number and complexity of public health emergencies involving the DGMQ over the past decade, the division's core funding has seen little increase. Rather than increased core funding, surge funding is appropriated for the DGMQ to access in times of emergency: This approach creates a cycle of boom and bust. Although surge funding has been critical to the DGMQ's response, it often comes too late to allow an efficient response, placing severe stress on existing staff. Because it is a temporary source of funding, there are limitations in how surge funding can be used and what type of personnel can be brought on board and supported. The division is in urgent need of more reliable funding streams than its traditional appropriations and intermittent surge funding. Current base funding is not commensurate with the DGMQ's responsibilities. Moreover, cycles of surge funding do not support a sustainable, proactive system that is ready to be deployed as soon as a public health emergency is identified. Consistent, reliable streams of funding are required to support this organization in fulfilling its mission of preparedness for public health emergencies.

Public health emergencies, most notably the COVID-19 pandemic, have strained an already limited workforce within the DGMQ. Although the number of approved full-time employee positions has increased since 2019, the majority of personnel at the DGMQ are currently in nonpermanent positions. Heavy reliance on temporary personnel poses several challenges, such as increased work for human resources (e.g., onboarding, badging, medical clearances), competition with other stakeholders for a limited pool of surge staff, and lower experience levels among staff. High vacancy rates among permanent positions have led to increased demands for overtime work, in turn resulting in burnout and high turnover. Combined with challenges in recruiting new hires, workforce issues are a vulnerability within the DGMQ. This is likely to affect not only the functioning of the division but is also likely to impact the culture and morale of the permanent staff. Leveraging technology and different recruitment methods may help meet increased workforce demands. Additionally, assessing the culture of the DGMQ could also address issues of burnout and provide means of supporting staff to reduce turnover.

> Recommendation 2-1: The U.S. Department of Health and Human Services (HHS), especially including the Centers for Disease Control and Prevention (CDC), should ensure that the Division of Global Migration and Quarantine (DGMQ) has the necessary financial and personnel resources, an effective organizational structure, and optimal infrastructure to effectively meet its responsibilities, execute its growing volume of work, and achieve its mission.
>
> To implement this recommendation, the DGMQ needs to specifically act and resolve the following issues:
> A. Organizational restructuring
>   1. Strong consideration should be given to restructuring the DGMQ to become a standalone unit with a direct reporting line to the CDC director.
> B. Finances
>   1. HHS should make a special agreement with the DGMQ to enable the DGMQ to utilize readily accessible funding in future emergencies. The process of acquiring and utilizing surge funds should be streamlined to facilitate greater flexibility during both their acquisition and during the drawdown period post-emergency.
>   2. The CDC should explore, along with the administration and Congress, the development of a user fee program to ensure that the division has a consistent and dependable source of revenue to cover the costs of operating quarantine stations.
> C. Workforce
>   1. The DGMQ should develop and implement a comprehensive and contemporary personnel plan to address multiple issues of recruitment, retention, skills development, vacancy rates, burnout, and excessive reliance on contract and temporary

staff. This plan should also include a commitment to diversity, equity, and inclusion, and to critical training needs and upskilling to prepare staff to successfully work in a dynamic, rapidly changing, and demanding environment and to stay abreast of evolving technologies. The plan should address the need for all quarantine stations to operate on a two-shift standard.
2. The DGMQ should develop and launch innovative strategies to support its critical recruitment needs.
    a. The organization should work with academic entities, such as universities and schools of public health, medicine, and law to develop a pipeline of future employees. Creative incentives and a streamlined human resources process should be used to facilitate the recruitment of graduates.
    b. The DGMQ should design, develop, and implement a "Ready Reserve Corps": a well-trained, experienced, and agile group of personnel with essential competencies who are preapproved and cleared, and thus could be immediately available to rapidly meet personnel needs of the organization during emergencies. This group should be paid a stipend to serve, be on standby status, and engage in training and practice exercises.
3. DGMQ should leverage opportunities presented through the CDC director's diversity, equity, and inclusion initiatives while undergoing the division's workforce study.

D. Culture
The DGMQ should assess its organizational culture and climate in association with the personnel and development plan to ensure that the division's values positively support its mission. This assessment should include a focus on diversity, equity, and inclusion. Corrective actions should be initiated if findings suggest that an adjustment is needed.

Recommendation 2-2: The Division of Global Migration and Quarantine (DGMQ) should create an effective and innovative quarantine-station model that matches the expanding and changing needs of a global, mobile world and augments its work in a progressively challenging infectious disease environment.

To achieve this recommendation, the DGMQ needs to implement these specific steps:
A. Develop criteria to determine whether a quarantine station should be added, deleted, or upgraded, and adjust the current number of stations accordingly. If a new station is deemed necessary, conduct

a business plan during preplanning to determine (1) the optimal number of staff to support a two-shift standard, (2) requisite staff competencies, (3) necessary support staff, and (4) capacity for routine round-the-clock coverage during emergencies if needed. If a new station is deemed necessary, conduct a business plan during preplanning to (5) determine whether the new site could have multiple uses and (6) identify potential partners that the new site could engage between and during emergencies. Finally, (7) adopt appropriate advanced technology including telemedicine options.

B. The maritime unit should be permanently housed within the DGMQ so that it can address the unique needs of the cruise industry and maritime-traveling public to enhance collaboration and disease control activities in maritime settings. The maritime quarantine station should have transparent operations and strong partnerships with regulated parties and other relevant entities.

C. Develop a more robust program for preclearance of passengers, immigrants, and animals, including collaborative actions with other pertinent agencies and organizations. The emphasis would be on upstream locations outside of the United States—to ease workload at entry sites.

D. Redesign post-entry follow-ups in partnership with local and state agencies, and other federal agencies, in which resources and responsibilities are better shared and modern technology is used for communications, tracking, and surveillance.

DISEASE CONTROL AND RESPONSE EFFORTS

Over the past two decades, the pace and variance of global infectious disease emergence has been accelerating at an alarming rate. This likely reflects a range of factors, including mass travel and migration, close animal/human interchange, and climate change. The DGMQ requires access to resources and tools for disease control that can be tailored to the specific threats. For individual travelers, the DGMQ's suite of infectious disease control tools includes travel restrictions—specifically the Do Not Board list, the Public Health Lookout, and (in conjunction with HHS and the White House) testing and/or vaccine requirements and restrictions on travel from particular countries experiencing infectious disease outbreaks.[1,2] In practice, these strategies have seen mixed success in mitigating disease spread.

Contact investigations are another tool used by the DGMQ to conduct

---

[1] This text was modified after release of the report to the study sponsor to correct the name of the list. Similar corrections have been made throughout the report.

[2] This text was modified after release of the report to the study sponsor to correctly describe the measures undertaken by DGMQ.

surveillance and protect the health of those who may have been exposed to infectious diseases during travel, with the aim of preventing further spread. When needed, the federal government can also exercise legal authorities to implement isolation and quarantine measures for individuals who may carry infectious diseases of high public health concern. As a federal agency, the DGMQ's powers are limited to those needed to prevent the entry of dangerous infectious diseases into the United States and to contain spread across state lines. DGMQ's mission is to prevent, detect, and respond to the spread of communicable diseases that impact the health of global and domestic travelers, migrants, immigrants, and refugees.

Considerations for ethics and equity must be central to the discussion of disease control measures—especially for interventions such as border closures and isolation and quarantine—and must take into account the variation in the types of travelers who enter the United States. For example, refugees and asylum seekers may need additional assistance to access services, and may be more vulnerable to consequences of border closures and travel restrictions. In addition to these core responsibilities related to international travelers, the DGMQ must respond to numerous other concerns. The DGMQ and CDC's Vessel Sanitation Program, run by the Center for Environmental Health,[3] interface with the maritime industry, responding to disease outbreaks on ships (cargo and cruise) at U.S. ports of entry. The DGMQ also regulates the entry of certain animals and products of animal origin into the United States and restricts animal products that could pose a public health risk.

The DGMQ was heavily involved in the COVID-19 response, collaborating with other CDC entities and other agencies to provide guidance on disease surveillance and mitigation, educate travelers, and work with various partners to implement public health measures. These experiences highlight the importance of scenario planning for the most likely and/or concerning potential disease outbreaks, with the active involvement of key partners. The committee found that the DGMQ could benefit from developing operational plans for emergency response based on lessons learned from recent disease events, such as SARS, MERS, Zika, influenza, COVID-19, and Ebola. The committee also found that disease control measures have not always maximized resource efficiency. For example, once COVID-19 transmission was widespread in the United States, quarantine and active monitoring of all international travelers coming into the United States—regardless of their symptoms or exposure history—was likely not effective in minimizing transmission in the country and diverted public health resources from other critical activities. These and other key lessons learned can be leveraged to guide policy decisions, such as travel restrictions and active

---

[3] This text was modified after release of the report to the study sponsor to correctly identify the entities responsible for responding to outbreaks at US ports of entry.

monitoring of international travelers to minimize risk of disease spread within the United States.

Recommendation 3-1: The Division of Global Migration and Quarantine (DGMQ) should develop detailed operational plans and playbooks based on the most concerning and likely scenarios for transmissible disease threats.
> A. The DGMQ should develop operational plans for the most probable scenarios that are likely to have major impacts requiring disease control interventions based on priority pathogens. These plans should list required partners, enumerate possible response steps, define possible implementation go–no go decision points, and include metrics to assess containment.
> B. The DGMQ should seek input from key agencies and organizations (e.g., the World Health Organization, the Coalition for Epidemic Preparedness Innovations, the U.S Agency for International Development, the new Centers for Disease Control and Prevention (CDC) Center for Forecasting and Outbreak Analytics, the CDC Center for Public Health Preparedness and Response, and the Office of the Assistant Secretary for Preparedness and Response) as well as state and local public health agencies when determining which pathogens and scenarios to prioritize for planning purposes.

Recommendation 3-2: The Division of Global Migration and Quarantine, in coordination with appropriate federal partners for implementation, should develop detailed operational plans for large-scale isolation and quarantine needs for future emergencies. These operational plans should be informed by the lessons learned during the initial response to COVID-19. Critical issues to address include:
> A. Potential sites for large-scale isolation and quarantine facilities should be identified in all Department of Health and Human Services regions. Memoranda of agreement for these facilities should be established prior to any possible need to facilitate rapid setup during a public health emergency. Minimum standards of infrastructure should be established for these facilities including capacity to provide wraparound services, such as health care services, diverse dietary needs, laundry facilities, communication needs, business support services, and entertainment.
> B. Ethical and equity issues that will likely arise, especially when housing/caring for special populations, including families with young children, the elderly, persons with special medical needs,

persons with disabilities, refugees, persons who cross borders on a routine basis for work, and persons with pets. The plans should also address language and incorporate intercultural components, normalizing these needs as an expected component of the public health response.
C. Those plans also need to include
1. coordination of legal authority and enforcement;
2. triage, transport, and assessment of ill persons with nearby health care facilities or onsite, available health care personnel; and
3. collaboration with state and local public health, law enforcement, and emergency management officials.

Recommendation 3-3: The Division of Global Migration and Quarantine/Centers for Disease Control and Prevention should commission an external formal evaluation and/or a modeling study of the effectiveness of travel restrictions and active screening/monitoring of all international travelers in preventing and mitigating disease transmission in the United States during both the current COVID-19 pandemic and the 2014–2015 Ebola outbreaks in West Africa. The formal evaluation should include psychological benefits, political implications, unintended consequences of screening, resources required, and burden placed on state and local jurisdictions. These findings should be used to inform plans detailing when such measures should be considered in the future and to specify the types of pathogens and scenarios that warrant these measures. The latter criteria might include incubation period, timing of infectiousness related to symptom onset, proportion of asymptomatic infections, size of traveler population that would require monitoring, technological ease and cost of monitoring, severity of illness, and reasonable ability to provide or implement countermeasures.

NEW TECHNOLOGIES AND DATA SYSTEMS

The DGMQ relies on technologies for disease mitigation, diagnostic testing, data collection, and communication. However, the COVID-19 pandemic has revealed striking inadequacies in the existing DGMQ technology infrastructure, even as the pandemic has resulted in the development and implementation of new technologies for health surveillance and communication. Innovative digital technologies for collecting and aggregating data are an essential tool for protecting public health from the introduction of diseases across international borders. These data are needed for contact tracing for individuals potentially exposed to infectious diseases, and for system reporting and monitoring and epidemic intelligence.

Technology can also be used to overcome limitations with staffing and to scale up, maximizing the effectiveness of screenings in airports and health departments. Contact tracing, for example, is more efficient when performed digitally rather than manually. However, major technical barriers of interoperability and standardization can limit the effectiveness of innovative digital tools to support the response to an infectious disease outbreak. Furthermore, there are some issues in legal, regulatory, and governance of data collection and sharing that can also pose a barrier to the adoption and effectiveness of innovative digital tools. Interoperability is critical for a strong and effective health care and public health system capable of flexing to respond to a public health emergency. Enhancing data interoperability can lead to improved early warning systems that integrate data from open sources as well as from traditional surveillance methods. Investments in data system interoperability can be lifesaving during a pandemic, improve day-to-day care coordination, and generate financial benefits to the United States. It is critical that the DGMQ update and improve its technology infrastructure in order to meet current and future demands during public health emergencies.

Clear, trustworthy public communication strategies are essential for explaining the need for digital technology, providing justification for the collection and use of personal data. As with all other aspects of disease control, ethics and equity must be central when considering and applying technology for disease mitigation. All technologies need to be used with safeguards for autonomy and privacy. Achieving this will require improved processes for data governance, such as through a CDC ethics committee or a DGMQ advisory committee.

> Recommendation 4-1: The Division of Global Migration and Quarantine (DGMQ) should increase and improve the use of innovative technology to aid in outbreak detection and response and to mitigate disease transmission. The DGMQ should improve readiness and develop flexible and targeted strategies for disease control at the border. The DGMQ should incorporate and improve on the use of digital technologies to gather health data from travelers, trace transmission, and alert travelers to exposures. These practices will also allow the development of scalable approaches to disease control strategies for large numbers of incoming travelers.

> Recommendation 4-2: The Division of Global Migration and Quarantine (DGMQ) should support the adoption of the Office of the National Coordinator for Health Information Technology (ONC) roadmap by health care and public health practitioners. The DGMQ should work with the ONC to facilitate the ONC roadmap and interoperability net-

works. Connectathons—events that allow providers, organizations, or other implementers to learn from developers, conduct testing, and practice exchanging data asynchronously across agencies—are an example of how this could occur. As health information technology developers continue to increase functionality in mobile health applications and electronic health records, the DGMQ should identify gaps and opportunities in legislation and regulation to support the proper use and transfer of information across data systems.

Recommendation 4-3: The Division of Global Migration and Quarantine (DGMQ) should ensure that all uses of digital technologies, novel data streams, and interoperative public health information systems follow a careful consideration of their ethical aspects and that all actions are in accordance with existing regulations for the protection of personal data. In order to achieve this, the DGMQ should put an oversight structure in place.

COORDINATION AND COLLABORATION

Partnerships are critical to the DGMQ's mission. The division works with both domestic and international partners in government and the private sector, including other nation's quarantine and disease control organizations; U.S. federal agencies; state, tribal, local, and territorial (STLT) agencies; and private-sector industries. One key example is the collaboration between the DGMQ and health officials in the United States and Mexico at various levels to (1) limit the cross-border spread of infectious diseases, (2) protect the health of people living in the U.S.–Mexico border region, and (3) promote the health of travelers, migrants, and other mobile populations. The DGMQ's success is highly dependent on its own capacity and that of its partners, including local public health departments and the U.S. Customs and Border Protection (CBP).

Coordination with travel industries is also an important example. The DGMQ's Quarantine Travel Epidemiology Team responds to reports of illness or exposure to disease that take place on airplanes, cruise ships, and cargo ships. The team works with state and local health departments, as well as with international partners, to facilitate contact investigations. This network of partnerships serves as the organizational and operational framework for implementing policies and activities to prevent and control the onward transmission of communicable diseases.

The COVID-19 pandemic has revealed opportunities to strengthen these relationships to facilitate coordination for future events. Making these relationships ongoing can help to ensure effective collaboration at the outset of an emergency. Regular engagement with jurisdiction-level stakeholders would facilitate clear and effective streams of communication. It will also be important to obtain perspectives from a broad range of stakeholders through a robust engagement process while policies are being developed and before they are finalized. Forming partnerships with academic institutions could also be helpful in analyzing the effectiveness of mitigation measures from previous public health emergencies to better understand the science behind the decisions including the economic cost of pandemic related measures.

> Recommendation 5-1: The Division of Global Migration and Quarantine (DGMQ) should strengthen partnerships through defined and planned activities that enhance working relationships and continue to build trust.
> To do so, the DGMQ should implement these specific measures:
> A. Improve collaboration with international partners through regularly scheduled forums:
>   1. Actively engage in the International Health Regulations (IHR) revision process.
>   2. Ensure the continuity of binational collaborations in border areas to facilitate the development of trust between partners. Participate with other agencies and partners in the development and implementation of a harmonized approach to border measures with Mexico and Canada that features common protocols for disease surveillance and response in border areas.
> B. Improve coordination between federal and state, tribal, local (county and city), or territorial (STLT) health agencies and strengthen international collaboration and engagement of quarantine officers.
>   1. Develop a Federal Interagency Workgroup with input from STLT partners.
>   2. Strengthen isolation and quarantine preparedness planning.
>   a. Define federal and STLT roles and responsibilities.
>   b. Understand and plan for variation in how STLT entities implement public health legal authorities.
>   c. Implement a federal and STLT tabletop exercise program to bring together relevant quarantine stakeholders to practice coordination periodically, especially in regions containing quarantine stations.
>   3. Ensure pre-decisional input and engagement from STLT health agencies. It is critically important that DGMQ guidance and documents are informed by ground-level local (county and city) health agencies.

a. Work to align DGMQ interventions with local public health activities to avoid overburdening the local public health system.
B. Improve coordination with aviation and maritime industries for border/traveler health issues and mandates:
   1. Build on coordination mechanisms established during the COVID-19 pandemic between aviation and maritime industries with STLT health agencies and the DGMQ. Examples of mechanisms for coordination include an Interagency Federal Workgroup, Memoranda of Agreement (MOA), Standard Operating Procedures (SOPs), emergency planning, drills, and exercises.
   2. Improve DGMQ engagement with regulated industries (e.g., cruise ship lines).
      a. Establish clear and consistent structure for communication.
      b. Develop clear objectives (e.g., safety and relative risk).
      c. Share and evaluate best practices at domestic and international ports.

Recommendation 5-2: The Division of Global Migration and Quarantine (DGMQ) should modernize health communication efforts with and for travelers to improve public understanding of disease control efforts as well as compliance.
A. Develop standardized communication for travelers, families of travelers, and the general public (e.g., what to expect when traveling to the United States) to ensure that travelers understand and change behaviors to follow disease control and prevention measures.
B. Establish mechanisms to utilize airlines, airport authorities, and travel agencies to communicate messages and better inform travelers during a pandemic, emerging pandemic, or outbreak.
C. Collaborate with the aviation industry to provide predeparture education and information sharing prior to flight boarding and during ticket purchase. Incorporate international best practices for communicating with passengers and sharing information regarding quarantine and testing requirements.
D. Incorporate avenues for the DGMQ to share informative materials with travelers in addition to the DGMQ website.
   1. Consider the use of electronic means of communication—such as flexible text messaging tools—to reach travelers with follow-up instructions and information.

E. In order to avoid health inequities, make these communications accessible for all travelers, regardless of language, access to technologies (e.g., smartphones), disabilities, and so on.

LEGAL AND REGULATORY AUTHORITY

The CDC has broad regulatory authority to control the introduction and interstate spread of communicable diseases in the United States. During the COVID-19 pandemic, the DGMQ has exercised powers granted to the CDC under the Public Health Service Act of 1944 (PHSA) by taking actions such as (1) testing, detaining, and releasing persons entering the United States who are suspected of carrying certain communicable diseases, (2) issuing federal isolation and quarantine orders, and (3) restricting importation of animals or other items that may pose public health threats. Examples of CDC orders enacted during the COVID-19 pandemic include Federal Quarantine and Isolation Order, No Sail/Conditional Sail Order, Global Testing Order, Safe Resumption of Global Travel, and the Face Mask Order. Many of these CDC actions were challenged in, or even blocked by, the courts. Reform of laws and regulations are needed to modernize the CDC's authorities, and to implement the committee's recommended measures on infrastructure, workforce, data systems, as well as important reforms to ensure it has the powers required to safeguard the American public.

Concerns related to CDC regulatory actions during the pandemic are primarily based on the interpretation of the PHSA, specifically the provision that grants the CDC the authority to take "necessary measures" to prevent the introduction into or spread of communicable diseases in the United States and across state borders. It will be critical for Congress to modernize the PHSA, which was enacted before the era of mass travel, migration, trade, and close animal/human interchange. The CDC will also need to undertake rulemaking to clarify its interpretation of the broadly delineated "necessary measures" provision and adopt procedural requirements and substantive standards to govern the use of its powers.

Also relevant to the use of regulatory power is the issue of DGMQ funding. Current large-scale funding methods for public health emergencies (PHEs) are inadequate. There are several options for expediting surge-funding mechanisms, such as (1) establishing a new PHE contingency fund that can be triggered under certain criteria during a PHE and (2) establishing a fund similar to the HHS Federal Emergency Management Agency (FEMA) Disaster Relief Fund.

Recommendation 6-1: Congress should improve the legal authority and flexibility of the Centers for Disease Control and Prevention (CDC) in

responding to public health threats by modernizing and improving the 1944 Public Health Service Act in several ways:
1. Give the CDC authority to effectively act to prevent or mitigate current and future public health threats. The CDC should have the authority it needs but must act consistently with scientific evidence, and only where necessary to prevent the interstate, intrastate, or international spread of infectious diseases. The CDC should also use the least restrictive alternative means that reasonably can be predicted to achieve an important public health objective.
2. Specifically delegate congressional power to reflect what the CDC needs to carry out its mission through evidence-based measures. These delegations should provide the CDC with robust authority and the necessary flexibility to implement science-based public health measures.
3. Include protections for individual rights and freedoms including procedural due process, where constitutionally warranted and feasible, to challenge any order under the Act.
4. Ensure that CDC authorities are fairly and equitably utilized.

REFERENCES

Barber, R. M., R. J. D. Sorensen, D. M. Pigott, C. Bisignano, A. Carter, J. O. Amlag, J. K. Collins, C. Abbafati, C. Adolph, A. Allorant, A. Y. Aravkin, B. L. Bang-Jensen, E. Castro, S. Chakrabarti, R. M. Cogen, E. Combs, H. Comfort, K. Cooperrider, X. Dai, F. Daoud, A. Deen, L. Earl, M. Erickson, S. B. Ewald, A. J. Ferrari, A. D. Flaxman, J. J. Frostad, N. Fullman, J. R. Giles, G. Guo, J. He, M. Helak, E. N. Hulland, B. M. Huntley, A. Lazzar-Atwood, K. E. LeGrand, S. S. Lim, A. Lindstrom, E. Linebarger, R. Lozano, B. Magistro, D. C. Malta, J. Månsson, A. M. Mantilla Herrera, A. H. Mokdad, L. Monasta, M. Naghavi, S. Nomura, C. M. Odell, L. T. Olana, S. M. Ostroff, M. Pasovic, S. A. Pease, R. C. Reiner Jr, G. Reinke, A. L. P. Ribeiro, D. F. Santomauro, A. Sholokhov, E. E. Spurlock, R. Syailendrawati, R. Topor-Madry, A. T. Vo, T. Vos, R. Walcott, A. Walker, K. E. Wiens, C. S. Wiysonge, N. A. Worku, P. Zheng, S. I. Hay, E. Gakidou, and C. J. L. Murray. 2022. Estimating global, regional, and national daily and cumulative infections with SARS-CoV-2 through Nov 14, 2021: A statistical analysis. *The Lancet*, April 8. https://doi.org/10.1016/S0140-6736(22)00484-6.

Institute of Medicine. 2006. *Quarantine stations at ports of entry: Protecting the public's health*. Washington, DC: The National Academies Press. https://doi.org/10.17226/11435.

Wang, H., K. R. Paulson, S. A. Pease, S. Watson, H. Comfort, P. Zheng, A. Y. Aravkin, C. Bisignano, R. M. Barber, T. Alam, J. E. Fuller, E. A. May, D. P. Jones, M. E. Frisch, C. Abbafati, C. Adolph, A. Allorant, J. O. Amlag, B. Bang-Jensen, G. J. Bertolacci, S. S. Bloom, A. Carter, E. Castro, S. Chakrabarti, J. Chattopadhyay, R. M. Cogen, J. K. Collins, K. Cooperrider, X. Dai, W. J. Dangel, F. Daoud, C. Dapper, A. Deen, B. B. Duncan, M. Erickson, S. B. Ewald, T. Fedosseeva, A. J. Ferrari, J. J. Frostad, N. Fullman, J. Gallagher, A. Gamkrelidze, G. Guo, J. He, M. Helak, N. J. Henry, E. N. Hulland, B. M. Huntley, M. Kereselidze, A. Lazzar-Atwood, K. E. LeGrand, A. Lindstrom, E. Linebarger,

P. A. Lotufo, R. Lozano, B. Magistro, D. C. Malta, J. Månsson, A. M. Mantilla Herrera, F. Marinho, A. H. Mirkuzie, A. T. Misganaw, L. Monasta, P. Naik, S. Nomura, E. G. O'Brien, J. K. O'Halloran, L. T. Olana, S. M. Ostroff, L. Penberthy, R. C. Reiner Jr, G. Reinke, A. L. P. Ribeiro, D. F. Santomauro, M. I. Schmidt, D. H. Shaw, B. S. Sheena, A. Sholokhov, N. Skhvitaridze, R. J. D. Sorensen, E. E. Spurlock, R. Syailendrawati, R. Topor-Madry, C. E. Troeger, R. Walcott, A. Walker, C. S. Wiysonge, N. A. Worku, B. Zigler, D. M. Pigott, M. Naghavi, A. H. Mokdad, S. S. Lim, S. I. Hay, E. Gakidou, and C. J. L. Murray. 2022. Estimating excess mortality due to the COVID-19 pandemic: A systematic analysis of COVID-19-related mortality, 2020–21. *The Lancet* 399(10334):1513-1536. https://dx.doi.org/10.1016/S0140-6736(21)02796-3.

1

Introduction

In an age of rapid global travel and escalating microbial threats, the importation of infectious pathogens of public health significance across national borders poses a substantial threat to the United States. The Centers for Disease Control and Prevention's (CDC's) Division of Global Migration and Quarantine (DGMQ) works to mitigate this threat by preventing the introduction, transmission, and spread of communicable diseases. This responsibility is complex and challenging, given that the United States typically receives nearly 1 million travelers per day across the nation's land, air, and sea ports of entry (CDC, 2021d). A cornerstone of the DGMQ's efforts to prevent the importation of infectious diseases among this high volume of incoming international travelers is its network of quarantine stations. As of March 2022, quarantine stations were located at 20 U.S. international airports and land-border crossings with the highest concentrations of arriving international travelers. Staffed with medical and public health officers, these quarantine stations are prepared to respond when ill travelers enter the country.

As the scope, volume, and frequency of microbial threats[1] have continued to intensify worldwide, the DGMQ has responded to an increasing number of infectious disease outbreaks over the past decade. Most notably, the COVID-19 pandemic—caused by severe acute respiratory syndrome

---

[1] For the purposes of this report, microbes include bacteria, viruses, protozoa, fungi, and prions that can replicate in humans (see the 2006 National Academies report *Quarantine Stations at Ports of Entry*, https://www.nap.edu/catalog/11435/quarantine-stations-at-ports-of-entry-protecting-the-publics-health, accessed May 19, 2022).

coronavirus 2 (SARS-CoV-2)—emerged as an outbreak in Wuhan, China, in December 2019. Declared a pandemic by the World Health Organization on March 11, 2020, an estimated 3.4 billion people have become infected with SARS-CoV-2 (Barber et al., 2022), resulting in over 18 million excess mortalities worldwide (Wang et al., 2022). COVID-19 has caused over 466 million confirmed cases and over 6 million deaths as of March 2022. The COVID-19 pandemic has starkly demonstrated the breadth of devastating health, social, and economic consequences that an infectious disease can wreak at a global scale. Moreover, it has highlighted the critical importance of identifying and implementing effective strategies and policies to mitigate the spread of infectious diseases of public health significance across national borders.

CHARGE TO THE COMMITTEE

The committee was charged with analyzing the effectiveness of the federal quarantine station network based on lessons from the COVID-19 pandemic. As specified in the committee's statement of task, the study was requested in order to (1) review how other relevant entities mitigate transmission risks for pathogens from arriving international travelers, (2) identify effective interventions, and (3) examine potential changes to the CDC's infrastructure and regulatory authorities. The committee was asked to review the DGMQ's current structure and function, including changes that have been made since the 2006 Institute of Medicine (IOM) report. It was also tasked with identifying how lessons learned during the COVID-19 pandemic and other public health emergencies can be leveraged to strengthen pandemic response. The committee's expertise comprised health law, ethics, behavioral science, health policy, state and local public health, medicine, global health, infectious diseases, health technology, and community health. The full statement of task for this consensus study is provided in Box 1-1.

This undertaking follows a 2006 IOM report, *Quarantine Stations at Ports of Entry: Protecting the Public's Health,* that had also been requested by CDC. The emergence of the COVID-19 global pandemic again prompted CDC to request that the National Academies of Sciences, Engineering, and Medicine convene a committee to conduct an external assessment of the role of DGMQ and the federal quarantine station network in mitigating the risk of onward communicable disease transmission in light of changes in the global environment, including large increases in international travel, threats posed by emerging infections, and the movement of animals and cargo.

INTRODUCTION

> **BOX 1-1**
> **Statement of Task**
>
> An ad hoc committee of the National Academies of Sciences, Engineering, and Medicine will assess the Centers for Disease Control and Prevention's (CDC's) Division of Global Migration and Quarantine (DGMQ) and the federal quarantine stations' strategies, policies, infrastructure, and resources dedicated to mitigating the risk of onward communicable disease transmission in the context of ongoing changes in the global environment, including large increases in international travel, threats posed by emerging infections, and the movement of animals and cargo. The committee will provide recommendations for the DGMQ to better respond to infectious disease outbreaks and pandemics. The committee will:
>
> 1. Review how other countries, international and multinational organizations and corporations, militaries with overseas operations, and other relevant entities mitigate transmission risks for pathogens like SARS-CoV-2 borne by arriving international travelers.
> 2. Identify effective interventions and best practices that could be adopted to the U.S.-specific context, recognizing challenges such as scale, data-gathering limitations, limited interoperability among partner networks, and the policy tools available to the CDC.
> 3. Examine potential changes to the CDC's infrastructure and regulatory authorities, to include:
>   a. How the DGMQ may leverage innovative approaches to data systems and/or analytical methods to mitigate scale limitations of the current process for implementing health screening and data collection at U.S. airports, and support health departments with post-arrival follow-up of travelers.
>   b. Potential changes to regulations that may be required to implement recommended measures.
>   c. The scope of responsibilities and types of partners needed at quarantine stations (such as state and local health officials), and how best to support these partners in preventing disease transmission in communities.
>   d. The relative importance of 24/7 coverage at high-traffic ports of entry versus adding more quarantine stations given budget constraints.
>   e. Optimal types of staff needed for CDC quarantine stations and at CDC headquarters.

Scope of Work

The committee worked to identify effective interventions and best practices for the context of a U.S.-specific response to a future pandemic. This involved consideration of the complexity and capacity restraints in mitigating disease introduction, safeguarding mobile populations and the travel industry, and implementing innovative data systems and analytics.

Such constraints include (1) scale limitations for health screening and data collection at U.S. airports; (2) challenges for gathering, analyzing, reporting, and validating data; (3) interoperability challenges between agency and partner networks in supporting public health; and (4) law and policy challenges related to the use of federal orders and the management of movement restrictions on large groups.

The committee reviewed needed changes in the CDC's infrastructure and regulatory authorities pertaining to

- how the DGMQ may leverage innovative approaches to data systems and/or analytical methods to mitigate scale limitations for current processes;
- potential changes to regulations to implement recommended measures;
- the scope of responsibilities and types of partners needed at quarantine stations;
- how best to support health departments and other partners in mitigating disease transmission; and
- optimal types of staff and scheduling at CDC quarantine stations and headquarters.

Study Methods

In developing this report and its recommendations, the committee deliberated for approximately 5 months, from November 2021 through March 2022. Their activities included four virtual meetings of 3 days each and one hybrid meeting of 2 days. Each of the virtual meetings included sessions open to the public; all public meeting agendas can be found in Appendix B. The committee's recommendations are directed at the CDC—specifically the DGMQ—and other stakeholders relevant to the Division's mission and operations.

The committee developed an approach for addressing each topic in the statement of task. Comparing international approaches to disease mitigation is an important item in the Statement of Task, and the National Academies commissioned a paper to be written that assessed a variety of disease control strategies implemented globally during the COVID-19 pandemic. International public health leaders were also invited to speak to the committee regarding COVID-19 mitigation measures implemented within their countries. Due to the context-specific nature of these measures and the committee's charge to develop recommendations specifically for the DGMQ, the committee decided not to include a detailed comparison of international approaches within this report, finding that this would detract from the focus of the report. Chapter 3 contains a description of the evidence presented for various disease control measures.

CURRENT FEDERAL QUARANTINE STATION NETWORK

Currently, the DGMQ operates a network of 20 quarantine stations located in U.S. ports of entry with high international travel volume. Notably, these stations are not physical areas through which incoming travelers pass into the United States. Rather, the term "quarantine station" refers to a group of individuals who perform activities designed to mitigate the risk of microbial and other threats of public health significance entering the United States (Institute of Medicine, 2006). Collaborating with other federal agencies such as Customs and Border Protection (CBP), the quarantine stations cover all 320 CBP U.S. ports of entry.[2] This report uses the term "port of entry" to mean any air, land, or seaport through which people, cargo, and conveyances may legally enter the United States from abroad.

The DGMQ is comprised of three branches: (1) Quarantine and Border Health Services; (2) Immigrant, Refugee, and Migrant Health; and (3) Travelers' Health; and two units: (1) United States–Mexico; and (2) Community Interventions for Infection Control. The Quarantine and Border Health Services Branch—one of the largest branches or units within the CDC in terms of number of federal employees and contractors—oversees 18 quarantine stations located within U.S. international airports as of March 2022 (Brown et al., 2021), The United States–Mexico Unit operates the two quarantine stations serving land-border crossings with Mexico. The stations are located in El Paso, Texas, and San Diego, California. Figure 1-1 depicts the geographic distribution of these quarantine stations across the United States. In addition to the 20 quarantine stations, the DGMQ operates three international field offices in Kenya, Thailand, and Mexico (CDC, 2021a).[3,4]

Expansion of the Quarantine Station Network

Almost a century after the first quarantine station was built at Philadelphia's port in 1799 after a yellow fever outbreak, the passage of the National Quarantine Act (1878) shifted some quarantine powers from the state to the federal level.[5] In 1944, the federal government's quarantine

---

[2] CBP's use of "port of entry" refers to an administrative center whose jurisdiction may include more than one entry facility in a certain geographic area (e.g., the Philadelphia Port of Entry services Philadelphia International Airport, Philadelphia's seaport, Trenton Mercer Airport, Atlantic City International Airport, and ports in Lehigh Valley, PA) (Institute of Medicine, 2006). Thus, the United States has over 470 literal ports of entry and 320 CBP ports of entry.

[3] More information about CDC quarantine stations can be found at https://www.cdc.gov/quarantine/quarantine-stations-us.html (accessed February 26, 2022).

[4] This text was modified after release of the report to the study sponsor to correctly reflect the number of international field offices.

[5] More information about the history of quarantine in the United States is available from https://www.cdc.gov/quarantine/quarantine-stations-us.html (accessed March 23, 2022).

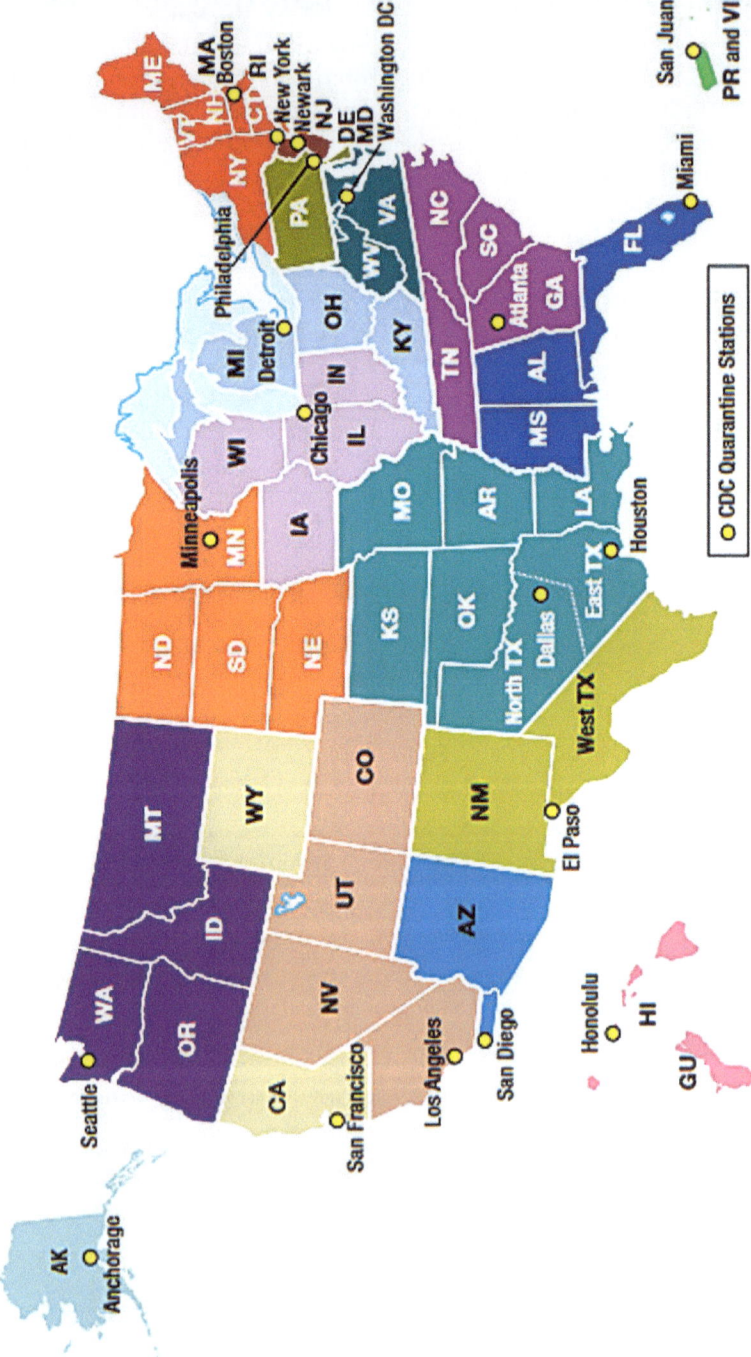

FIGURE 1-1 CDC quarantine stations and their jurisdictions.
SOURCE: CDC, 2021c. https://www.cdc.gov/ncezid/dgmq/pdf/Quarantine-and-Border-Health-H.pdf (accessed May 20, 2022).

power was codified in the Public Health Service Act of 1944 (PHSA) and, in 1967, the CDC's predecessor National Communicable Disease Center assumed federal quarantine functions. Throughout the 1970s, the CDC's network of quarantine stations was reduced from more than 50 to fewer than 10 based on the presumption that infectious diseases no longer posed a major public health threat. However, anthrax attacks using contaminated letters (2001) and a severe acute respiratory syndrome (SARS) outbreak (2003) renewed concerns about bioterrorism and infectious disease threats and catalyzed the expansion of the federal quarantine station network. In fiscal year 2003, Congress began allocating funds for an expansion to a total of 25 quarantine stations at ports of entry including airports, seaports, and land-border crossings (Institute of Medicine, 2006).

Prior to 2004 the network consisted of quarantine stations located at eight international airports—New York (JFK), Miami, Chicago, Los Angeles, Atlanta, San Francisco, Honolulu, and Seattle—with limited staffing. In 2005, the network expanded to include quarantine stations at the airports in Washington, DC; Houston; Newark; Boston; Detroit; Minneapolis; Anchorage; and San Juan; two stations serving U.S.–Mexico land-border crossings were also created that year in El Paso and San Diego. In 2007, spurred by an IOM consensus study report, quarantine stations in Philadelphia and Dallas were added to the network. The report also recommended five additional locations in Charlotte, New Orleans, Phoenix, Denver, and Kansas City, but those have not yet been established. Thus, the number of quarantine stations increased by almost three-fold in 3 years—from 8 in 2004 to 20 in 2007—but no new quarantine stations have been established since 2007.

The DGMQ's network of quarantine stations is responsible for executing a range of activities to protect the public's health at U.S. ports of entry by rapidly responding to sick travelers who arrive in the United States, alerting travelers about disease outbreaks, and restricting the importation of animals and products that may carry disease. The key roles and responsibilities of DGMQ quarantine stations are outlined in Box 1-2. Among those roles is the delegated authority to implement isolation and quarantine for individuals under specific circumstances. Isolation separates individuals who are proven or highly suspected of being sick with a designated infectious disease of consequence from individuals who are not sick. Quarantine separates and restricts the movement of people who were exposed to an infectious disease to see if they become sick. Although quarantine and isolation functions at national borders are critical tools for limiting the importation and spread of infectious disease threats, their effectiveness varies based on the type of threat and the extent of its current spread (Institute of Medicine, 2006).

> **BOX 1-2**
> **Roles and Responsibilities of DGMQ Quarantine Stations**
>
> - Responding to reports of illnesses and deaths on airplanes, ships, and at land-border crossings
> - Planning and preparing for emergency response
> - Responding to mass migration emergencies
> - Inspecting animals, animal products, and human remains that pose a potential threat to human health
> - Inspecting CDC-regulated cargo and hand-carried items for potential vectors of human infectious diseases
> - Building partnerships for disease surveillance and control
> - Creating partner training materials for station staff to use during their on-site trainings of port and public health partners
> - Supporting health monitoring and collecting medical information of new immigrants, refugees, asylees, and parolees, when needed
> - Providing travelers with essential health information
> - Distributing immunobiologics and medications under investigational new drug protocols (currently intravenous artesunate and antitoxins for botulism and diphtheria).
>
> SOURCE: https://www.cdc.gov/quarantine/quarantine-stations-us.html (accessed March 16, 2022).

The federal government has legal authorities[6] to implement isolation and quarantine measures to help prevent the public's exposure to an individual who has or may have specific infectious diseases of great public health risk (CDC, 2021b). An executive order by the president authorizes federal isolation and quarantine for a specific set of infectious diseases; this list can also be revised by the president through executive order. Currently, isolation and quarantine are federally authorized for cholera, diphtheria, infectious tuberculosis, plague, smallpox, yellow fever, viral hemorrhagic fevers (i.e., Lassa, Marburg, Ebola, Crimean-Congo, South American, and others not yet isolated or named), SARS, influenza caused by novel or

---

[6] The authority for isolation and quarantine derives from the Commerce Clause of the U.S. Constitution. Under section 361 of the Public Health Service Act (42 U.S. Code §264), the U.S. Secretary of Health and Human Services is authorized to take measures to prevent the entry and spread of communicable diseases from foreign countries into the United States and between states. Isolation and quarantine also are considered "police power" functions that are derived from the state's right to take action affecting individuals for the benefit of society. (Source: https://www.cdc.gov/quarantine/aboutlawsregulationsquarantineisolation.html; accessed March 15, 2022.)

reemergent influenza viruses that are causing—or have the potential to cause—a pandemic, and measles (CDC, 2021b).

The U.S. Department of Health and Human Services (HHS) has delegated its federal authority[7] to carry out isolation and quarantine functions to the CDC. Thus, if an individual who arrives at a U.S. port of entry—via air travel, maritime travel, or land-border crossing—has a suspected or confirmed case of a designated quarantinable infectious disease, quarantine station staff have the delegated authority to detain, medically examine, or conditionally release that individual. The CDC's authority to order that such individuals be medically evaluated can supersede the public health powers of states and localities under specific circumstances (Institute of Medicine, 2006). However, despite these authorities, the CDC has traditionally deferred to state and local public health officials to implement isolation and quarantine in such instances. During the outset of the COVID-19 pandemic, however, the CDC implemented isolation and quarantine for individuals entering the United States from Hubei Province, China, and two cruise ships with identified outbreaks (CDC, 2020).[8]

2006 IOM REPORT AND SUBSEQUENT DEVELOPMENTS

The 2006 IOM consensus study report *Quarantine Stations at Ports of Entry: Protecting the Public's Health* provided a set of recommendations about how the DGMQ's quarantine station network could strengthen its capacities to mitigate disease importation and its response to infectious threats at the nation's borders (Institute of Medicine, 2006). Key recommendations from that report include

- increasing U.S. efforts and providing sufficient financial resources to minimize microbial threats from travelers;
- working with partners to harmonize authorities for sufficient contact data;
- enhancing the competencies, number of staff, space, and technological capacity of the quarantine stations with an expansion to 25 stations;
- conducting periodic review of processes and optimal locations of quarantine stations;

---

[7] Under 42 Code of Federal Regulations parts 70 and 71, the CDC is authorized to detain, medically examine, and release persons arriving into the United States and traveling between states who are suspected of carrying these communicable diseases. (Source: https://www.cdc.gov/quarantine/aboutlawsregulationsquarantineisolation.html; accessed March 15, 2022.)

[8] This text was modified after release of the report to the study sponsor to correctly reflect and specify where isolation and quarantine orders were implemented.

- developing proper surge capacity for emergencies with deployment of CDC assets and hiring plans, including locations for isolating travelers and communication plans to interface with health care staff and media;
- developing a research agenda to examine basic public health interventions for use in the system; and
- developing scientifically sound tools to measure the effectiveness and quality of operations at the quarantine stations.

In response to these recommendations, the DGMQ increased the ability to conduct risk assessment for microbial threats. The DGMQ also developed a series of tools and practices including a data system to catalogue all events occurring at quarantine stations and support follow up activities for ill travelers, such as documenting diagnostic test results. However, post-arrival public health follow-up has been limited due to failure to implement an electronic traveler contact data collection system.[9] In addition to expanding the number of quarantine stations in the network, the stations have been revamped in response to the recommendations made in the 2006 report. However, not all of the other recommendations have yet been incorporated due to a decision to instead expand additional international locations. Offices in Kenya, Thailand, and Mexico were established to support these activities.

In its work, this committee was asked to further identify effective interventions and best practices to mitigate disease introduction into the United States. This undertaking involves consideration of numerous challenges specific to developments since the 2006 report was published. Chapter 2 outlines the increased responsibilities outbreak mitigation efforts have entailed in recent years. Over the past decade, regular emergencies have become part of normal operations—see Figure 2-2. This reflects a greater need to build preparedness into the structure of the DGMQ. Although operating costs have risen dramatically since 2014, the majority of this funding has come from response-specific and reimbursable funds, while programmatic core funds have been slow to increase. Furthermore, the DGMQ's staffing needs have grown considerably. While permanent full-time employee positions have seen only modest growth since 2008, the total full-time equivalent—which includes contractors and other nonpermanent positions—has grown more than five-fold in the same time period (Damon, 2022). This study assesses the DGMQ and its needs in the context of the frequent emergence of disease threats.

The COVID-19 pandemic has presented myriad challenges and involved large-scale isolation and quarantine response efforts, some of which

---

[9] This text was modified after release of the report to the study sponsor to correctly describe the tools and practices used by the DGMQ.

had never before been implemented. The committee reviewed the effectiveness of these efforts and highlighted lessons yielded from the pandemic response. They also explored the proliferation of technological developments that have emerged since the 2006 report in order to recommend strategies to leverage and optimize current capabilities.

This study also takes into account critical issues regarding ethics and equity that must be considered when developing and implementing a public health response to emerging threats—particularly given the rapid advancement of technological innovations for disease surveillance and mitigation as well as the existing inequities that have been highlighted by the COVID-19 pandemic. It is increasingly imperative to employ measures that do not further exacerbate these inequities. Ethical risks must also be considered when designing infectious control strategies, especially those that employ novel, powerful digital technologies and data systems. To guide its deliberations, the committee identified a set of key ethical principles: (1) protecting privacy, (2) maintaining autonomy, (3) promoting equity, (4) minimizing the risk of error, and (5) ensuring accountability.

The global impact of the COVID-19 pandemic revealed the broad range of partners with which the DGMQ must engage to effectively execute its roles and responsibilities in mitigating transmissible disease threats, including federal interagency partners; state, tribal, local, and territorial agencies; international partners; and private-sector entities. This study highlights the critical importance of fostering trust and strengthening the DGMQ's functional working relationships across agencies and sectors to effectively counter future infectious disease threats.

Additionally, the COVID-19 pandemic demonstrated that public health authority designated by legislation enacted before the age of large-scale global travel needs to be modernized. Thus, the committee has recommended a set of policy changes to expand authorities and streamline funding for emergency events.

STRUCTURE OF THE REPORT

This report is organized to reflect five primary factors that determine the effectiveness of the federal quarantine station network, as identified by the statement of task and the expert committee. These factors are organizational capacity; disease control and response efforts; new technologies and data systems; coordination and collaboration; and legal and regulatory authority. Chapter 2 provides an overview of the organizational capacity of the DGMQ, highlighting key issues surrounding workforce, financials, infrastructure, and culture within the division. Chapter 3 describes the DGMQ's role in infectious disease control and provides an assessment of various disease mitigation measures. Chapter 4 describes the technology that has been implemented by the DGMQ and details innovations developed during the COVID-19 pandemic—both in the United States and abroad—that can be adopted to increase the DGMQ's capacity for surveillance and data sharing. Chapter 5 describes the partnerships with federal, state, and local health authorities that the DGMQ relies on to fulfill its mission. Chapter 6 offers a detailed analysis of the legal and regulatory framework that underpins the DGMQ's authority, addressing mechanisms for modernizing applicable public health response powers.

REFERENCES

Barber, R. M., R. J. D. Sorensen, D. M. Pigott, C. Bisignano, A. Carter, J. O. Amlag, J. K. Collins, C. Abbafati, C. Adolph, A. Allorant, A. Y. Aravkin, B. L. Bang-Jensen, E. Castro, S. Chakrabarti, R. M. Cogen, E. Combs, H. Comfort, K. Cooperrider, X. Dai, F. Daoud, A. Deen, L. Earl, M. Erickson, S. B. Ewald, A. J. Ferrari, A. D. Flaxman, J. J. Frostad, N. Fullman, J. R. Giles, G. Guo, J. He, M. Helak, E. N. Hulland, B. M. Huntley, A. Lazzar-Atwood, K. E. LeGrand, S. S. Lim, A. Lindstrom, E. Linebarger, R. Lozano, B. Magistro, D. C. Malta, J. Månsson, A. M. Mantilla Herrera, A. H. Mokdad, L. Monasta, M. Naghavi, S. Nomura, C. M. Odell, L. T. Olana, S. M. Ostroff, M. Pasovic, S. A. Pease, R. C. Reiner, Jr., G. Reinke, A. L. P. Ribeiro, D. F. Santomauro, A. Sholokhov, E. E. Spurlock, R. Syailendrawati, R. Topor-Madry, A. T. Vo, T. Vos, R. Walcott, A. Walker, K. E. Wiens, C. S. Wiysonge, N. A. Worku, P. Zheng, S. I. Hay, E. Gakidou, and C. J. L. Murray. 2022. Estimating global, regional, and national daily and cumulative infections with SARS-CoV-2 through Nov. 14, 2021: A statistical analysis. *The Lancet*, April 8. https://doi.org/10.1016/S0140-6736(22)00484-6.

Brown, C., F. Alvarado-Ramy, and A. Klevos. 2021. *To screen or not to screen? There's more to border health than interventions at our borders: CDC*. Presentation to the National Academies of Sciences, Engineering, and Medicine Committee on Analysis to Enhance the Effectiveness of the Federal Quarantine Station Network.

CDC (Centers for Disease Control and Prevention). 2020. *CDC issues federal quarantine order to repatriated U.S. citizens at March Air Reserve Base* [Media Statement]. https://www.cdc.gov/media/releases/2020/s0131-federal-quarantine-march-air-reserve-base.html (accessed May 18, 2022).

CDC. 2021a. *Laws and regulations*. Division of Global Migration and Quarantine (DGMQ). https://www.cdc.gov/ncezid/dgmq/laws-and-regulations.html (accessed May 18, 2022).

CDC. 2021b. *Legal authorities for isolation and quarantine*. https://www.cdc.gov/quarantine/aboutlawsregulationsquarantineisolation.html (accessed March 15, 2022).

CDC. 2021c. *Quarantine and border health services*. Division of Global Migration and Quarantine (DGMQ). https://www.cdc.gov/ncezid/dgmq/focus-areas/quarantine.html (accessed February 28, 2022).

CDC. 2021d. *Who we are*. Division of Global Migration and Quarantine (DGMQ). https://www.cdc.gov/ncezid/dgmq/who-we-are.html (accessed February 25, 2022).

Damon, J. 2022. *Review of budget and staffing—DGMQ funding, staffing, and turnover data 2019–2021: CDC*. Presentation to the National Academies of Sciences, Engineering, and Medicine Committee on Analysis to Enhance the Effectiveness of the Federal Quarantine Station Network.

Institute of Medicine. 2006. *Quarantine stations at ports of entry: Protecting the public's health*. Washington, DC: The National Academies Press. https://doi.org/10.17226/11435.

Wang, H., K. R. Paulson, S. A. Pease, S. Watson, H. Comfort, P. Zheng, A. Y. Aravkin, C. Bisignano, R. M. Barber, T. Alam, J. E. Fuller, E. A. May, D. P. Jones, M. E. Frisch, C. Abbafati, C. Adolph, A. Allorant, J. O. Amlag, B. Bang-Jensen, G. J. Bertolacci, S. S. Bloom, A. Carter, E. Castro, S. Chakrabarti, J. Chattopadhyay, R. M. Cogen, J. K. Collins, K. Cooperrider, X. Dai, W. J. Dangel, F. Daoud, C. Dapper, A. Deen, B. B. Duncan, M. Erickson, S. B. Ewald, T. Fedosseeva, A. J. Ferrari, J. J. Frostad, N. Fullman, J. Gallagher, A. Gamkrelidze, G. Guo, J. He, M. Helak, N. J. Henry, E. N. Hulland, B. M. Huntley, M. Kereselidze, A. Lazzar-Atwood, K. E. LeGrand, A. Lindstrom, E. Linebarger, P. A. Lotufo, R. Lozano, B. Magistro, D. C. Malta, J. Månsson, A. M. Mantilla Herrera, F. Marinho, A. H. Mirkuzie, A. T. Misganaw, L. Monasta, P. Naik, S. Nomura, E. G. O'Brien, J. K. O'Halloran, L. T. Olana, S. M. Ostroff, L. Penberthy, R. C. Reiner, Jr., G. Reinke, A. L. P. Ribeiro, D. F. Santomauro, M. I. Schmidt, D. H. Shaw, B. S. Sheena, A. Sholokhov, N. Skhvitaridze, R. J. D. Sorensen, E. E. Spurlock, R. Syailendrawati, R. Topor-Madry, C. E. Troeger, R. Walcott, A. Walker, C. S. Wiysonge, N. A. Worku, B. Zigler, D. M. Pigott, M. Naghavi, A. H. Mokdad, S. S. Lim, S. I. Hay, E. Gakidou, and C. J. L. Murray. 2022. Estimating excess mortality due to the COVID-19 pandemic: A systematic analysis of COVID-19-related mortality, 2020–21. *The Lancet* 399(10334):1513-1536. https://dx.doi.org/10.1016/S0140-6736(21)02796-3.

2

Organizational Capacity

Organizational capacity (OC) is the ability of an organization to perform work and ensure that its organizational resources are used effectively and efficiently to achieve its goals. In the context of governmental organizations, OC is a multidimensional concept that refers to the organization's ability to marshal, develop, direct, and control its financial, human, physical, and information resources. OC captures the collective skills, abilities, knowledge, and experiences of an organization.

Various models for conceptualizing OC have been proposed, but almost all include four key features: infrastructure, finances, workforce, and culture (Cox et al., 2018). These four elements, which are evaluated in this chapter, represent the means and mechanisms through which the people and resources in an organization are brought together and utilized to accomplish its work, achieve its goals, and fulfill its mission. Like any organization, OC underpins and shapes the identity and personality of the Centers for Disease Control and Prevention's (CDC's) Division of Global Migration and Quarantine (DGMQ). Thus, as the key determinant of the DGMQ's performance, OC is essential to understanding the organization's effectiveness, its efficacy, and its ability to execute tactics and strategies aligned with its intentions and purpose.

The DGMQ's infrastructure is central to its OC and is a key element in protecting public health as people become increasingly mobile within today's globally interconnected world. Financial management involves the deployment of funds and other assets to achieve organizational goals. More specifically, it entails budget planning, acquiring funds, distribution, and allocation of resources. The domain of workforce and human resources includes personnel recruitment, retention, training, development, competencies, and performance. Finally, culture encompasses an organization's values, norms, behaviors, and beliefs. Culture is integral to both individual and collective performance within an organization, as well as its ability to be adaptive and remain relevant. Although culture is difficult to measure, it often serves as the glue that holds an organization together (Cox et al., 2018).

Throughout the extraordinary work environment of the last decade, the DGMQ has continued to evolve in the face of complex challenges stemming from our global interconnectedness, the speed of travel and trade, and the integration of unprecedented societal changes, especially those resulting from the COVID-19 pandemic. Despite the advances made, the DGMQ faces significant challenges that undermine its ability to fulfill its mission. With core funding that has remained inadequate over the last decade, the division is limited in its ability to keep pace with a regular stream of public health emergencies. Persistent understaffing and burnout demonstrate the institutional challenges. The DGMQ must undergo significant changes with its finances, workforces, and culture in order to become a more agile and responsive structure. It must be successful in this formidable and disruptive setting, but achieving this will require absorbing, adapting, and being able to pivot quickly. The pillars of OC are foundational in helping the organization improve its work and performance. Without significant and rapid changes, the DGMQ's capacity to lead the nation in preparedness and response is severely limited.

Much of the information in this chapter was provided by DGMQ representatives during open public committee meetings. Because detailed information about infrastructure, workforce, finances, and culture is not available from other publicly available sources, these presentations were invaluable in allowing the committee to assess the inner workings of the DGMQ and develop salient conclusions and recommendations. These four critical areas of OC reflect the evidence presented to the committee and, while critical, are not exhaustive. Other aspects of organizational capacity may warrant further exploration.

DGMQ INFRASTRUCTURE

The DGMQ works to maintain public health security by preventing the introduction, transmission, and spread of infectious diseases into the United States within a context of rapid global travel.[1] The DGMQ is one of the nine offices and divisions housed within the National Center for Emerging and Zoonotic Infectious Diseases (NCEZID). The NCEZID collaborates with national and global partners to mitigate the impact of infectious

---

[1] More information about the DGMQ's work is available from the CDC (2016).

diseases (CDC, 2016). The DGMQ's primary functions include screening, processing, and evaluating travelers—including immigrants and refugees—entering the country for any public health risks, and providing them with public health information. The DGMQ partners with airlines and cruise lines to identify sick travelers and alert other passengers of potential exposure. The division forwards information to local public health officials to enable individual follow-up and collaborates with these officials to prevent people with certain infectious diseases from traveling and exposing others. The DGMQ is also tasked with regulating the entry of animals, processing animal imports, and restricting animal products harmful to human health. Additionally, the division is responsible for emergency distribution of essential drugs and biologics, such as botulism antitoxin, under CDC investigational new drug (IND) protocols. In addition, the DGMQ periodically distributes investigational drugs of critical public health importance under IND when commercially available drugs are ineffective or have had supply disruptions, such as intravenous artesunate for severe malaria. Quarantine stations began stocking this drug when the CDC received U.S. Food and Drug Administration (FDA) approval to distribute it in 2007 for patients who failed treatment with intravenous quinidine (the only FDA-approved drug for severe malaria), then expanded distribution in 2019 after quinidine was no longer available in the United States (Rosenthal and Tan, 2019).[2] This section provides an overview of the composition and function of the DGMQ's infrastructure, with a particular focus on the Quarantine and Border Health Services Branch (QBHSB) and the network of quarantine stations operated by the DGMQ.

Quarantine Stations and International Field Offices

The United States receives nearly 1 million travelers per day across the nation's land, air, and sea ports of entry (CDC, 2021d). To prevent the spread of contagious diseases into the United States, the CDC DGMQ operates 20 quarantine stations as of March 2022. Most stations are located within U.S. international airports with the highest volumes of arriving international travelers; two stations are located at U.S.–Mexico land-border crossings, which handle approximately 25 percent of daily legal land crossings. The QBHSB oversees the 18 airport-based quarantine stations, while the San Diego and El Paso land border stations fall under the purview of the United States–Mexico Health Unit. Each station has its own jurisdiction, which includes the various subports such as seaports, land-border crossings, and smaller airports within a geographic area. Collaborating with

---

[2] This text was modified after release of the report to the study sponsor to provide additional clarity about DGMQ activities under the CDC's investigational new drug protocols.

other federal agencies, such as Customs and Border Protection (CBP), the quarantine stations cover all (> 300) U.S. ports of entry.[3]

In addition to those 20 quarantine stations, the DGMQ currently operates three international field offices in Kenya, Mexico, and Thailand (Cetron, 2021).[4] The offices in Kenya and Thailand primarily support activities undertaken by the Immigrant, Refugee, and Migrant Health Branch while the Mexico Office supports activities undertaken by the U.S.–Mexico Unit for populations moving back and forth across the U.S.–Mexico border or residing in the border region (Institute of Medicine, 2006).

Structures of Quarantine and Border Health Services Branch and the United States–Mexico Unit

Headquartered in Atlanta, the QBHSB is among the largest branches within the CDC in terms of its number of federal employees and contractors (Brown et al., 2021). As illustrated in Figure 2-1, the branch includes five teams that report directly to the U.S. QBHSB branch chief: (1) the Quarantine Travel Epidemiology Team (QuarTET); (2) the Epidemiology Field Team (eFIT), (3) the Zoonoses Team (ZTeam); (4) the Preparedness and Policy Coordination Team (PPCT); and (5) the Communication, Evaluation, and Training (ComET) Team. In addition to these teams, the QBHSB has a chief medical officer who oversees surveillance and clinical activities, and makes recommendations on overall detection and control strategy. The deputy branch chief supervises the Resource Support Services Team (RSST) and the Operations Team. Branch operations include managing the 18 quarantine stations, which are subdivided into four regions, each of which has a regional officer in charge. The chief medical officer and deputy branch chief report directly to the branch chief.

The QBHSB houses the principal activities related to quarantine station operations. QuarTET supports response to ill travelers. This includes managing implementation of federal public health travel restrictions (Do Not Board and Public Health Lookout).[5] QuarTET also facilitates response to exposures to communicable diseases of public health concern during air and maritime travel and coordinates contact investigations with federal, state, tribal, local, and territorial (STLT), and international partners. QuarTET provides guidance, trainings, and standard operating procedures so that staff at quarantine stations can respond appropriately. The eFIT is

---

[3] See https://www.cbp.gov/border-security/ports-entry#:~:text=Locate%20Port%20Information,of%20entry%20throughout%20the%20country (accessed May 20, 2022).

[4] More information about CDC quarantine stations can be found at https://www.cdc.gov/quarantine/quarantine-stations-us.html (accessed February 26, 2022).

[5] More information about federal public health travel restrictions is available from https://www.cdc.gov/quarantine/do-not-board-faq.html (accessed February 24, 2022).

ORGANIZATIONAL CAPACITY

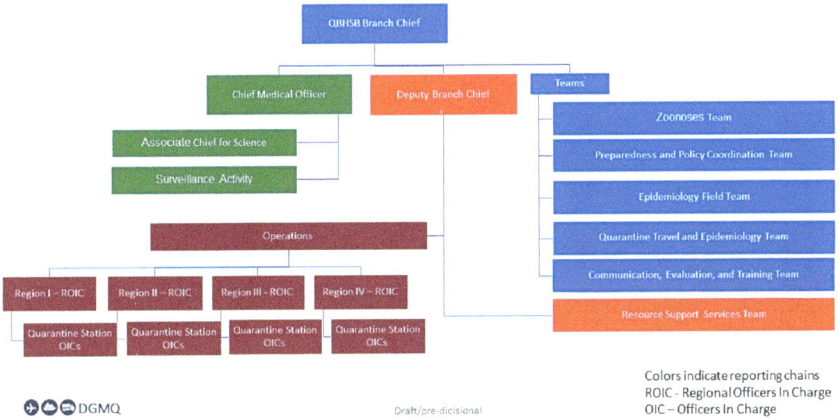

FIGURE 2-1 Organizational chart, Quarantine and Border Health Services Branch (QBHSB).
SOURCE: Brown et al., 2021, slide 8.

composed of a cadre of epidemiologists that carry out projects to advance the science and practice of travel and border public health. The ZTeam works to prevent the introduction and spread of diseases from imported live animals, animal products, or human remains by administering, and updating when needed, the CDC's regulatory authorities and issuing guidance. Recent areas of focus for this team include canines, nonhuman primates, and mink (and mink products). The PPCT is responsible for preparedness planning for hazards and continuity of operations, emergency operations and response management, and preparedness training. The team also analyzes travel data, develops exercises, and facilitates and evaluates the development of After Action and Improvement Plans. Additional focus areas include quarantine station operations support and SharePoint site development and management. The ComET team works to train branch personnel and is responsible for communicating health information through various mechanisms, including posters, handouts, websites, and media responses. The RSST provides logistical support for operations at the quarantine stations.

The United States–Mexico Unit (U.S. MU) oversees the land ports of entry along the 2,000-mile U.S.–Mexico border. General protocols and training are derived from the QBHSB, but adapted for land border–specific environments. The permanent quarantine station staff and surge contractors located in San Diego and El Paso respond remotely to illnesses, exposures, and importations at all land ports of entry on the U.S.–Mexico border. Also housed within the U.S. MU is the Mexico Country Office, the Border Epidemiology Unit focused on strengthening U.S.–Mexico border state surveillance and response, and the Migrant/Communications team with specific activities for mobile southern border populations. Together, the QBHSB and the U.S. MU manage the quarantine station network with support from the DGMQ's Office of the Director.

Recent Responses to Disease Threats

The DGMQ is responsible for preventing the importation and spread of a number of disease threats. Daily quarantine station operations include restricting the importation of animals and animal products that may carry disease and containing the importation and spread of pathogens—such as rabies and monkeypox—from animals or vectors. The stations respond to ill travelers who arrive in the United States, along with addressing communicable disease case-patients (e.g., tuberculosis [TB], measles) or outbreaks (e.g., varicella, SARS-CoV-2).[6] During outbreaks of infectious diseases of concern in other countries, the division works to protect travelers and contain the importation and spread of pathogens from specific locations or regions into the United States. For example, during the Ebola virus disease epidemic in Western Africa (2014–2016), the DGMQ recommended that Americans avoid nonessential travel to the three countries most affected by the epidemic. Working with airports and federal authorities, the division streamlined response efforts by diverting passengers from countries experiencing outbreaks to five U.S. airports. The division also trained U.S. Customs and Border Protection staff at airports to screen these passengers for symptoms of Ebola or possible exposures (CDC, 2021b). During the Zika virus disease outbreaks in the Americas (2015–2016), the DGMQ focused efforts on traveler education and outreach, especially for pregnant travelers and their partners. Outreach efforts included posted travel notices about preventing the spread of Zika, interactive maps, risk assessment tools, text messaging systems, and extensive airport messaging. Quarantine stations located in areas that were at greater risk of Zika spread, such as the U.S.–Mexico border and Puerto Rico, built partnerships with local governments and community health workers to alert travelers about Zika risk (CDC, 2021b).

Public health emergencies of international concern as declared by the World Health Organization (WHO)[7]—such as polio and the COVID-19 pandemic—fall under the DGMQ's purview. In 2009, the CDC (including the DGMQ) collaborated with state and local health departments to stop the spread of the H1N1 influenza pandemic in the United States (CDC,

---

[6] This paragraph was modified after release of the report to the study sponsor to correctly characterize some of DGMQ's responsibilities. Similar corrections have been made throughout the report.

[7] For more information on public health emergencies of international concern and the CDC, see: https://www.cdc.gov/nndss/about/ihr.html (accessed May 3, 2022).

2021b). In 2020, the CDC began its largest and most complex response to date in addressing the COVID-19 pandemic. The DGMQ's efforts focused on protecting travelers and other mobile populations and reducing the risk of importing and spreading COVID-19 by way of global travel. Activities included

- taking regulatory actions, such as no-sail orders, quarantine measures for incoming international travelers, mask requirements on public transportation, and a rental eviction moratorium;
- establishing public health guidance for managing infected travelers and travelers potentially coming from countries deemed at greater risk due to high countrywide transmission levels;
- publishing travel guidance and health notices;
- establishing and conducting public health entry screening; and
- providing refugees, immigrants, and migrant workers with culturally and linguistically appropriate resources related to COVID-19.

Additional DGMQ efforts focus on controlling communicable disease outbreaks at immigration detention centers and repatriation locations. For example, the DGMQ issued quarantine orders for U.S. citizens repatriated from Wuhan, China, and cruise ships that were affected by initial outbreaks of COVID-19 in early 2020 (CDC, 2021b). This responsibility has also included responses to COVID-19 outbreaks at U.S. southern border locations. The division also addresses communicable diseases associated with mass migration emergencies, such as the displacement of Afghan refugees in 2021 and 2022 (Roohi, 2022). These actions complement those of the Department of Homeland Security, which establishes entry requirements for incoming travelers at U.S. ports of entry (Department of Homeland Security, 2022).

Infrastructure Challenges and Constraints

The responses to disease threats required thus far in the 21st century reflect the challenges the DGMQ faces in carrying out its mission. The division is involved in frontline activity in the majority of CDC disease threat responses, yet it lacks efficient mechanisms to quickly surge staff. Responsibilities have been increasing with each response, and the DGMQ is dependent on supplemental funding to carry these out, as discussed in the next section. The ability to urgently scale up health screening and data collection at U.S. airports in the immediate response to a newly emerging disease threat is limited, and challenges in gathering, analyzing, reporting, and validating data are at play. There are also challenges in ensuring effective coordination with STLT partners to manage both cases and exposed passengers when they leave the airport or cruise ship. The division is considering how innovative approaches to data systems or analytical methods might be leveraged to mitigate these scale limitations (see Chapter 4). However, the scope of responsibilities for quarantine stations and the types of partners needed to meet them are broad. Furthermore, interoperability issues between agency and partner data systems pose challenges to unified public health efforts. The DGMQ is one of the few organizational components at the CDC with regulatory responsibilities, which places an added burden on the division and requires unique skill sets such as regulation writing and legal support. Managing movement restrictions of large groups of people—and using federal orders to do so—poses policy, operational, and legal challenges. Thus, the implementation of recommended measures may involve changes to regulations governing the CDC's and DGMQ's activities and authorities (see Chapter 6).

High Traveler Volume across Numerous Border Entries

International experts from South Korea, Hong Kong, Canada, Taiwan, Singapore, Australia, and the United Kingdom spoke to the committee regarding their countries' procedures for screening, isolation, and quarantine of incoming passengers during the COVID-19 pandemic (see Chapter 3). Notable differences between the United States and other nations were apparent. A primary difference is that the volume of incoming passengers to other countries is much lower than the volume arriving in the United States. Moreover, many of the countries represented at the briefings (Taiwan, Australia, Canada) closed their borders to most incoming individuals when the COVID-19 pandemic began, whereas the United States primarily closed its borders to individuals traveling from specified high-risk regions (Hoffman and Poirier, 2022). The number of entry points is also much smaller in these other countries than in the United States and were further restricted during the COVID-19 pandemic. Whereas many countries had few points or only a single point of entry, the United States has approximately 320 land, air, and sea border entry points (Buigut and Maskery, 2021). Also, many of these presenters represented island nations, making access easier to restrict. Effectiveness of entry requirements and containment measures is highly dependent on context, making comparison between countries challenging.

In spite of the large number of U.S. points of entry, only 20 of them contain quarantine stations (CDC, 2021c), resulting in approximately 300 border entry points without any consistent public health service presence on site (CDC, 2021c). These border crossings may have a limited need for public health assistance and are staffed by other federal agencies. The 20 quarantine stations are strategically positioned at border entries with high concentrations of international travelers (See Chapter 1). Approximately 80 percent of all international arrivals enter the United States via an airport with an associated quarantine station (CDC, 2019a).[8] However, public health threats can appear at any border entry point, so there is a need to expand the CDC presence to the other ports of entry (Walls, 2021). Therefore, solutions, including enhanced capacity for telehealth, are needed to assure adequate availability of public health services for personnel at all border crossings at all times.

Pandemic-Related Demand Increases

Other challenges relate to pandemic-related demand increases. In recent years, the DGMQ has been active in simultaneous responses, which can prove taxing for staff. For example, from 2020 to 2021, the division addressed Ebola virus disease outbreaks, concerns on the Southwest border due to the large number of persons arriving for immigration into the United States, the evacuation of Afghan refugees, and the COVID-19 pandemic. Screening processes established to address COVID-19 increased demands on the DGMQ. For instance, the number of individuals screened for COVID-19 across 15 designated U.S. airports rose from less than 1,000 on March 11, 2020, to nearly 30,000 by March 14, a mere 3 days later (Buigut and Maskery, 2021; Dollard et al., 2020).

The scale of demands posed by the COVID-19 pandemic is highlighted when comparing it with the Ebola epidemic of 2014 to 2016. The latter involved the screening of more than 38,000 travelers entering the United States in a span of 16 months (Cohen et al., 2016). In contrast, more than 760,000 travelers were screened for COVID-19 at U.S. airports in only 7 months (January–December 2020) (Dollard et al., 2020). Once Ebola data collection efforts began, the CDC was able to share contact data for all travelers with STLT public health agencies who were tasked with monitoring over 99 percent of them, post-arrival. In the first 7 months of the COVID-19 pandemic, contact data for 32 percent of screened travelers could not be shared due to data collection limitations. Many states opted out of receiving data due to the fact that STLT health officials were focused on addressing known COVID-19 cases and contacts rather than screening all travelers, most of which were at low risk of illness or exposure. The monitoring rate for travelers for COVID-19 after arrival is unknown.

The DGMQ is already among the largest and most complex divisions within the CDC and needs to grow. It has a unique set of responsibilities and is one of the few units at the CDC with direct regulatory responsibilities. It is also one of the few CDC components that operates field units,

---

[8] This text was modified after release of the report to the study sponsor to correctly reflect the percentage and type of travel.

including those with international responsibilities. Other federal agencies, such as the U.S. Department of Agriculture (USDA), have successful overseas preclearance programs that increase work efficiency at U.S. ports. The DGMQ presently has overseas personnel stationed in Kenya, Thailand,[9] and Mexico. However, today's public health emergencies and refugee crises can emerge in almost any part of the world. Developing a more robust overseas presence could enable earlier and more effective response efforts. In addition, a pre-identified and cleared team of experts could be established, allowing them to be deployed when needed if there is an emerging threat from a specific region. While not specifically studied by the committee, there may be merit in redesigning the organization to include a more unified network of quarantine stations and functions.

Maritime Unit

The current structure of the maritime unit poses unique logistical challenges. Prior to the COVID-19 pandemic, two distinct CDC entities addressed maritime public health. The Maritime Activity, housed under the DGMQ, liaised with quarantine stations regarding communicable diseases of public health concern on maritime vessels, developed procedures for quarantine stations, and supervised management of outbreak response on vessels. The Vessel Sanitation Program (VSP), housed under the National Center for Environmental Health, managed cases of gastroenteritis on cruise ships. In April 2020, these entities merged to form a temporary Maritime Unit under the Global Migration Task Force. While the formation of the Maritime Unit has allowed for enhanced cooperation in responding to public health concerns on maritime vessels, challenges have emerged with the transition. As this merging was intended to be a temporary solution, the Maritime Unit is not permanently housed within any division (Tardivel, 2022). As gleaned from stakeholder presentations during committee meetings, there has been a perception among some stakeholders of a lack of communication between the Maritime Unit and the cruise industry, contributing to frustration regarding clarity in regulations and requirements from industry. Establishing a permanent base for the Maritime Unit could allow for improved communications, enhanced recruitment efforts, and greater effectiveness in achieving public health goals.[10]

---

[9] Kenya and Thailand were selected as base locations for DGMQ's Africa and Asia Field Programs (respectively), which oversee medical screening for immigrants and refugees traveling to the United States (see https://www.cdc.gov/ncezid/dgmq/focus-areas/irmh.html; accessed March 10, 2022).

[10] See Chapter 3 for additional information on the Maritime Unit, including disease control strategies.

DGMQ'S FINANCIAL LANDSCAPE

Trends in the DGMQ Budget and Allocations (Fiscal Years 2012–2022)

The committee was briefed on trends in budgeting and allocations to the DGMQ and its quarantine stations over the past decade (Damon, 2022).

Baseline Funding

The DGMQ's aggregated core budget lines—that is, its usual operating budget—supports its mission and programmatic activities. A substantial proportion of the DGMQ's core funding also supports the salary and benefits for DGMQ permanent staff responsible for executing mission and programmatic activities (Cetron, 2021). The DGMQ's baseline funding saw little to no increase over the past decade, despite substantial increases in the DGMQ's responsibilities and the growth of international travel during that period (Cetron, 2021). Between fiscal year (FY) 2012 and FY2022, the DGMQ's core funding has remained relatively static year over year, except for a small increase in FY2020's core ceiling (Damon, 2022). Baseline funding has remained between $45–54 million per year, with an average increase each year of just 1 percent. The budgeting and allocation trend remained particularly flat for the salary and benefits for DGMQ permanent employees during that period.

Response Surge Funding

The DGMQ has received supplemental funds to support additional activities required during emergency responses. For instance, surge funding has been implemented during emergencies such as the COVID-19 pandemic. Emergencies that resulted in influxes of supplemental response-specific funding prior to the COVID-19 pandemic include the Ebola virus disease epidemic (Western Africa) (FY2014–FY2016) and the Zika virus disease epidemic in the Americas (FY2016–FY2017) (Damon, 2022). Thus, individual public health response supplemental funds have shaped the DGMQ's budgetary trends over the past decade. Between FY2012 and FY2022, the DGMQ's total budget fluctuation year over year has been strongly response driven, with a significant driver of the DGMQ's current operating budget being its near-constant state of emergency response (see Figure 2-2). There is a need for an accessible central emergency fund that can be readily accessed in the event of emergencies to prevent delays in financing critical response elements (see Chapter 6). Surge funding has been a lifeline to the DGMQ and its ability to address emergencies. However,

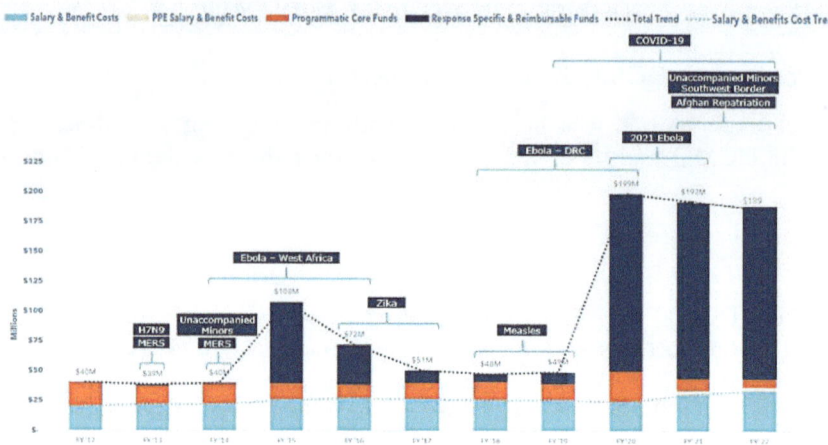

FIGURE 2-2 DGMQ's 10-year budget trends.
NOTE: The budget is largely response driven, with a notable increase for fiscal year 2020–2022.
SOURCE: Damon, 2022, slide 79.

whether funding will be allocated, the amount of funding, and its timing are uncertain in the early phases of the response. The funds often come late in a response and because surge funding is temporary, there are limitations in how it can be used; usually only temporary or contractual personnel can be brought on board and supported using these funds.

Added Responsibilities and Activities

Each new public health emergency brings additional responsibilities for the DGMQ, placing further strain on its infrastructure, finances, and workforce. To support this expanded work, the DGMQ allocates a larger percentage of its core operational funding to support salary and benefits. This requirement decreases the remaining funding within the core budget to conduct mission and programmatic activities. Although the salary and benefits proportion of core funding has increased year over year between FY2012 and FY2022, baseline funding has remained static (Damon, 2022). For FY2021 and FY2022, 2-year limited COVID-19 funding is being used to support the salary and benefits for 24 permanent positions provided to the DGMQ in the agency's FY2021 Enterprise Hiring Plan. Once the limited COVID-19 funding ends, other funds will need to be used to support these full-time equivalents (FTEs).

With the COVID-19 pandemic response (FY2020–FY2022), the DGMQ has executed close to $200 million annually (discussed in further detail in the next section). The DGMQ projects that the long-term impacts

ORGANIZATIONAL CAPACITY 43

of the pandemic will include an expanded DGMQ work portfolio that includes regulatory actions taken to mitigate the burden of COVID-19. The result is a new permanent staffing requirement to support expanded regulatory and programmatic work and increased programmatic costs to sustain mission activities. In light of this, leadership within the DGMQ and the CDC supported a congressional appropriation request to increase the DGMQ core funding by $30 million (Damon, 2022). The FY2022 appropriation ultimately included an $8 million increase to the DGMQ's core funding. However, this anticipated core funding increase in budget comes almost 3 years into the pandemic and remains a critical need that has not been addressed swiftly enough.

High-Level Overview of the DGMQ Budget: Fiscal Year 2021 and 2022

The committee was provided with a high-level overview of the DGMQ's budget for FY2021 and FY2022, including funding streams in aggregate—reflecting both proposed and anticipated increases—as well as categories in which funding is spent, and program spending power at current core funding levels (Damon, 2022).

Funding Streams

The DGMQ's two major funding streams include core funding and supplemental response allocations. The division received almost $192.1 million in total obligated funding in FY2021, with a reduction to $189.7 million proposed for FY2022. Core funding had nearly $45.1 million obligated in FY2021, with a 1.5 percent increase planned for FY2022, bringing the total core funding to about $45.8 million. The FY2022 President's Budget request proposed $30 million increase to the DGMQ's core budget will be critical to sustain its mission and programmatic activities. As previously described, significant DGMQ activities are funded through response supplemental funding lines. The DGMQ supplemental response allocations had about $146.4 million obligated in FY2021 and $143.3 million planned for FY2022. The CDC has proposed an $8 million increase in response allocations for FY2022 (Damon, 2022).

Spending Categories

Of the almost $192.1 million in total funding (including supplemental funds) obligated to the DGMQ in FY2021, virtually all of the funds went to three categories: contracts (61 percent), grants and cooperative agreements (21 percent), and salary and benefits (17 percent). For FY2022, there is a planned salary and benefits increase of 15 percent to support infrastructure priority positions. However, the DGMQ's core funding increase is just 1.5 percent from FY2021 to FY2022, so the planned salary and benefits increase of 15 percent will require a decrease in the DGMQ's mission and program spending from core funding.

DGMQ spending on grants, cooperative agreements, and contracts will remain fairly constant in FY2022 relative to FY2021. Grants and cooperative agreements may increase by $2.4 million (a 6 percent increase). However, grants and cooperative agreements are primarily supported through supplemental funding. They also reflect the DGMQ's partnership engagements and collaborations to support public health interventions and improve the effectiveness of interventions. The spending on contracts will stay largely the same between FY2021 and FY2022, with a slight decrease in contracts of $9.4 million (8 percent decline) (Damon, 2022). This reflects the DGMQ operating infrastructure required to execute both mission and programmatic activities as well as response-related work.

Spending Power

DGMQ program spending power at current core funding levels is directly impacted by the need for increased staffing to sustain its mission and programmatic activities. In FY2021, 65 percent of the core funding ceiling ($45.1 million) was spent on salary and benefits, leaving 35 percent of that funding to cover all operational and programmatic costs, including mission and regulatory activities. Based on the planned core funding ceiling for FY2022 ($45.8 million) and given the planned increase to salary and benefits, about 74 percent of funding will be spent on salary and benefits, leaving just 26 percent to sustain operational, mission, and regulatory activities.

Hypothetical Financing Scenarios for Fiscal 2023

The committee heard two hypothetical financing scenarios for FY2023. If the DGMQ's needs are not prioritized financially, the staffing footprint required to facilitate its preparedness for public health emergencies and to fill all authorized positions would leave no funds remaining for program and mission work.

Specifically, for FY2023, core funding projected at current levels will be about $46.4 million—all of which will need to be spent on salary and benefits, leaving no core funding for programmatic, mission, and regulatory efforts and nonpersonnel operational costs. If the proposed $30 million FY2022 increase to core funding is realized, however, the core ceiling will increase to about $76 million. This will enable 67 percent of core funding to cover salary and benefits, with 33 percent for programmatic, mission, and regulatory work. Although the anticipated increase to its core funding would allow the DGMQ to hire to its approved staffing level, it would merely be able to sustain—but not grow—its programmatic and mission work.

These two hypothetical scenarios are untenable. Therefore, it is clear that the DGMQ requires additional funding. A permanent income stream beyond congressional funding could be one means of achieving this. Baseline core funding has been flat for years and has left permanent staffing underfilled. The reliance on surge funding in crises is unsustainable for meeting consistent staffing requirements. The establishment of a "no year" emergency response fund, with sufficient funds to cover crisis activities and increased surge staff needs, would obviate the wait for annual congressional appropriations and supplemental appropriations in crisis situations.

Potential Funding Streams

Currently, the DGMQ does not have sufficient core funding to support its personnel and programs. Increased core funding is needed to sustain programmatic activities so the organization does not have to rely solely on emergency funding that is only made available at some point after the start of an emergency (see Chapter 6). The DGMQ could explore sources of funding in addition to the standard congressional appropriation to support its core personnel and activities. For instance, the DGMQ could explore whether user fees—from industries that receive direct benefit from DGMQ activities and regulatory oversight such as the maritime and aviation industry—could provide a sustainable source of funding. The CDC's VSP, in which cruise industries pay user fees to have their vessels inspected, sets precedent for this arrangement (CDC, 2019b). User fee charges could be tied to objective criteria such as the number of passengers per year. A caveat is the potential for a conflict of interest on the part of the DGMQ, as it would be paid by the industries being regulated. Although this practice is somewhat controversial, other federal agencies have successfully implemented similar strategies (FDA, 2022). The division is in need of other more reliable funding streams besides its traditional appropriations and surge funding. The committee is aware that there may be barriers to establishing user fee authority; however, in other agencies, user fee programs have been transformative in improving staffing and program performance. Since the DGMQ performs an array of critical, direct services at the border that support regulated industries and the public, there is an adequate basis for such a funding mechanism. There is also a need for better human resources (HR), thereby allowing for more nimble hiring of personnel to fulfill surge needs. Current staff are now absorbing the workload of the vacant unfilled positions, contributing to substantial levels of burnout.

WORKFORCE

Over the past decade, the DGMQ has been operating in emergency response mode more often than not. Therefore, operating in response mode has become the de facto normal operational state and tempo, not be viewed as unusual or the exception. However, both its number of FTE employees and its level of core funding have remained nearly unchanging despite the escalating size of the DGMQ's suite of responsibilities. Currently, surge responses to emergencies are being managed as individual, time-limited occurrences. They are supported by temporary funding and large numbers of temporary personnel and staff. This short-term solution does not effectively address the division's long-term needs. It is imperative that the DGMQ, including its quarantine stations, be appropriately staffed to fulfill its mission and execute its responsibilities.

Trends in DGMQ Staffing Requirements and Levels

Within the DGMQ, the number of permanent, FTE employees has remained static for years (Damon, 2022). However, between FY2019 and FY2022, the response to the COVID-19 pandemic has generated a substantial increase in staffing needs. To meet these needs, the DGMQ has used term-limited federal appointees (TERM NTE), training program appointments, and contractors. Note that all federally appointed employees worked full time and that TERM NTE only indicates the distinction between term-limited and permanent employees. To meet mission and regulatory requirements, this increase in staffing has involved slow upscaling through resource-intensive recruitment and hiring, as well as the use of contract mechanisms (Figure 2-3).

Evaluation of DGMQ Staffing Composition: 2019–2022

The committee was provided with a high-level overview of the evolution of the DGMQ's total staffing composition—including both permanent and nonpermanent staff types—between FY2015 and FY2022 (Damon, 2022). Nonpermanent staff types include malaria-funded TERM NTE positions (hired prior to the COVID-19 response for expanded distribution of intravenous artesunate under the CDC's investigational new drug protocol), COVID-19–funded TERM NTE positions, contractors, fellows, students, and guest researchers. Authorized permanent staffing levels[11] remained relatively static from FY2015 to FY2019, maintaining approximately 180 FTE

---

[11] The authorized permanent staffing level does not represent an occupancy rate. Although authorized, not all permanent positions were filled during these fiscal years.

positions. By FY2019, the number of approved positions in the DGMQ increased to 223 FTE positions, however, the DGMQ did not have the core funding to fill and maintain this permanent staffing footprint. Thus, the DGMQ has compensated with an enhanced footprint of TERM NTEs, contractors, fellows, and other nonpermanent employee types.

Between FY2019 and FY2022, there was a marked escalation in overall staffing resources. In FY2022, the number of approved FTE staff positions in the DGMQ increased to 331 (Damon, 2022). This was catalyzed by (1) multiple ongoing responses, (2) expanding regulatory requirements, and (3) increasing mission activities inclusive of response efforts. With a continued lack of core funding, the DGMQ has continued with an enhanced nonpermanent staffing footprint.

The escalation in overall staffing from FY2019 to FY2022 was also driven by increases in temporary staffing to support the response to the COVID-19 pandemic. During that period, the number of authorized TERM NTE positions increased almost seven-fold, from 17 to 115. During the same period, the staffing ceiling for contractors and fellows spiked 32-fold from 24 to 770 positions. By FY2022, the DGMQ had an unprecedented number of positions for TERM NTEs, contractors, fellows, and other employee types. Thus, the overall volume of temporary staffing dwarfed the volume of permanent staffing by roughly four-fold in FY2022. Positions held by TERM NTEs, contractors, and fellows have increased from 41 in 2019 to 885 in 2022 to support the DGMQ's response, mission, and program requirements (Damon, 2022).

For over a decade, the DGMQ has had a chronic deficit in baseline funds (see previous section). This deficit has not permitted the division to keep pace with its growing responsibilities and work effectively in an era of unprecedented infectious disease emergencies. The DGMQ's non-emergency workload has concurrently grown due to significant increases in international travel and trade, migration, and population relocations. The division is in the unenviable position of determining whether to use funds to support personnel or programmatic activities, as there is not enough funding to do both. The DGMQ has received additional FTEs. But if they use their funds to support these FTEs, there will be no remaining funds to support program activities. This is analogous to a "fool's choice" as both are imperative to fulfill their mission.

Current DGMQ Staffing, Occupancy, and Turnover Rates

The division has more than 1,100 permanent and nonpermanent positions currently staffed, although this number is consistently in flux. Nonpermanent staff currently comprise a significant proportion (77 percent) of the total staff.

Occupancy and turnover rates among DGMQ staff remain major ongoing concerns. In FY2019, the DGMQ's average occupancy rate for FTE positions was about 82 percent, which declined to 77 percent in FY2022 (Damon, 2022). The volume of staff leaving DGMQ has also increased sharply in recent years. In FY2021, the DGMQ saw significant turnover of 44 FTE staff lost; although they were able to maintain staffing at a level near that of 2020 by bringing on 44 new staff, there was no net gain (Damon, 2022). From 2019 to 2021, there was an increase in the turnover of employees leaving the DGMQ by approximately two-fold (Damon, 2022). Most departures were among staff in the general schedule (GS)-9 and GS-11 (mid-level) categories, with a noticeable shift toward those staff leaving the agency entirely rather than staying within the CDC. The committee did not explore staffing trends across the CDC but, if similar, the CDC may benefit from an agencywide approach to rebuilding the workforce.

Quarantine and Border Health Services Branch Staffing Levels

Based on FY2022 staffing levels, the QBHSB is the fourth-largest branch at the CDC in terms of the number of federal staff—including FTE and TERM NTE staff—and the second-largest branch at the CDC if contractors are included (Brown et al., 2021). Figure 2-3 illustrates the overall trends in total staffing for QBHSB between 2008 and 2022, including both authorized and filled positions for FTE staff, TERM NTE staff, contractors, students, training programs, and deployers (the CDC and the Department of Health and Human Services [HHS] staff that are deployed to assist in the DGMQ work). Spikes in the numbers of nonpermanent staff—particularly contractors—correlate directly with major response efforts, including the influenza A (H1N1) pandemic (2009), the Ebola virus disease epidemic in West Africa (2014–2016), the Zika virus disease epidemic (2015–2016), the expansion of distribution of the intraveinous artesunate for severe malaria (2019), and the COVID-19 pandemic (2019–2022).

As of November 2021, there are currently 252 approved positions within the DGMQ's QBHSB, including 108 approved FTE positions and 144 TERM NTE positions (Brown et al., 2021). The overall vacancy rate for both FTE and TERM NTE staff is about 42 percent (November 2021), with 146 of 252 total approved positions filled (Brown et al., 2021). The vacancy rates are widely variable (0–60 percent) across the five in-house teams that report directly to the QBHSB branch chief: ZTeam, 60 percent vacancy rate (4/10 approved positions filled); QuarTET, 50 percent (17/34); PPCT, 30 percent (7/10); eFiT, 29 percent (5/7); ComET, 0 percent (7/7). Additionally, nearly half of the QBHSB Operations Team (the quarantine stations) positions are currently vacant (86/160), but almost all of the ap-

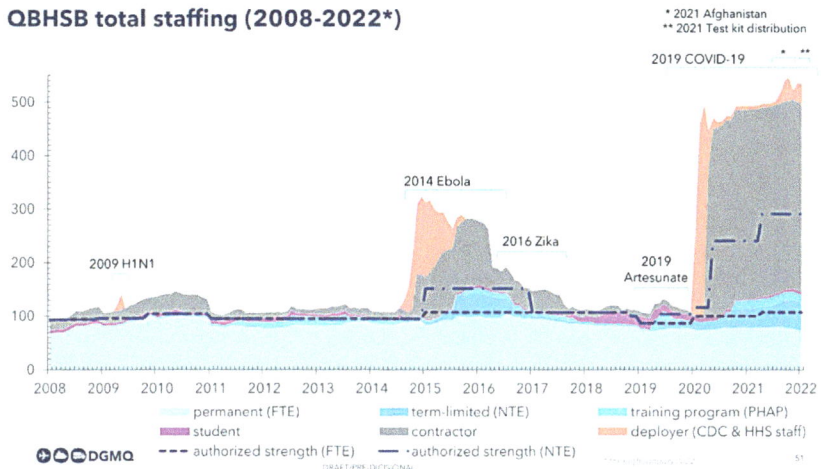

FIGURE 2-3 Quarantine and Border Health Services Branch (QBHSB) total staffing, 2008–2022.
NOTES: CDC = Centers for Disease Control and Prevention; FTE = full-time equivalent (permanent staff); HHS = Department of Health and Human Services; NTE = temporary federal appointees; PHAP = Public Health Associate Program.
SOURCE: Alvarado-Ramy, 2022, slide 51; based on data from QBHSB consolidated staffing records.

proved positions at QBHSB Headquarters are filled (10/11) and most of the Resource Support Services Team positions are filled (10/13).

Quarantine Station Staffing Levels

As of March 2022, the DGMQ operates 20 designated quarantine stations (18 airports and 2 land border crossings) (CDC, 2022). As conveyed by discussions with DGMQ representatives during committee meetings, the number of positions at each of the quarantine stations is determined by multiple factors: (1) volume of arriving international travelers, immigrants, and refugees; (2) cargo volume (especially for primate, canine, and other CDC-regulated importations); (3) geographic coverage and risk factors specific to the jurisdiction of quarantine station (including the number and types of ports of entry within the jurisdiction and number of arrivals from high-risk geographic areas); (4) number of responses occurring at a given time; and (5) the availability of cross-station coverage for surges in operations (CDC, 2021a).

Among the 18 quarantine stations located at international airports in the network, there are currently 160 approved positions—the majority of which are TERM NTE positions. The number of total approved positions at each quarantine station varies widely, from 4 each at the Anchorage and

Philadelphia stations, to 16 at the New York station located in John F. Kennedy airport (Brown et al., 2021). Overall, only 86 (54 percent) of these approved positions were occupied as of November 2021, representing a total vacancy rate of 46 percent (Brown et al., 2021). The vacancies are most glaring for the TERM NTE appointments, of which just 41 of 104 positions (39 percent) are occupied, versus 45 of 56 (80 percent) FTE positions.

Like the number of positions, the vacancy rates vary widely across the network of quarantine stations, from 25 to 75 percent as of November 2021 (Brown et al., 2021). Vacancy rates at some of the larger stations are noteworthy: San Francisco Quarantine Station (67 percent), Atlanta Quarantine Station (60 percent), Los Angeles Quarantine Station (40 percent), and New York Quarantine Station (44 percent). The lowest vacancy rates are at the Philadelphia Quarantine Station (25 percent), Chicago Quarantine Station (31 percent), and Washington, DC Quarantine Station (33 percent). The current staff per station currently ranges between 1 and 9 individuals, which contrasts sharply with the range in the number of approved positions across the stations (4–16 positions).

Workforce Challenges

The DGMQ's primary workforce-related challenges include lack of sufficient funding to support adequate staffing, understaffing of permanent and temporary positions, and high rates of vacancy and turnover.

Funding Challenges

As previously described, the DGMQ received a substantial increase to its permanent staffing footprint in FY2022. Unfortunately, the division has not received a commensurate increase to its core funding to sustain the expansion to the staffing ceiling and maintain program activities. Thus, the increase in the DGMQ's permanent staffing ceiling represents a driver for the decreased spend power of the DGMQ's core budget. Moreover, the regular budget process has not provided a sufficiently sustainable source of funding for permanent staff. Instead, there have been periodic infusions of emergency funding which cannot be used to support long-term, permanent staff (see Figure 2-2).

The committee was provided with a breakdown of how authorized staffing ceilings within the DGMQ were funded in FY2019 versus FY2022 (Damon, 2022). During FY2019 all 223 authorized FTE positions were supported by core funding. In FY2022, the same number of FTE positions were also funded by the core, despite the authorization of an additional 108 permanent positions. Of those additional positions, 91 have a response supplemental temporary source of funding to support the position through the end of that fiscal year, while 17 do not have an identified source of funding.[12] In FY2019, all 17 TERM NTE positions were supported by core funding; in FY2022, all 115 temporary positions were supported by supplemental response funding. The 24 positions for contractors and fellows were entirely core funded in FY2019. In FY2022, 735 of the 770 positions for contractors and fellows were funded by response supplemental funding lines, while 35 were supported by core funding.

Challenges in Recruiting and Retaining Permanent Staff

The DGMQ currently relies heavily on TERM NTE staff, contractors, and fellows—as opposed to permanent staff—in order to execute its responsibilities, but this is inadequate and inefficient for operating with and sustaining long-term effectiveness. Required competencies, including skill sets and qualifications, within these nonpermanent categories of personnel may be limited or not appropriately aligned to the position or job requirements they are expected to perform. In addition, term positions are established using emergency funds, which means the positions are dissolved once the emergency is over unless alternative funding and positions are identified. This is not a sustainable model for a functional organization. This manner of staffing in the DGMQ not only affects the division's efficiency and functionality but can also undermine employee morale. An additional inefficiency of temporary personnel is high turnover, resulting in the loss of acquired organizational knowledge. Temporary personnel and contractors may also not be as committed to the culture and success of the organization as permanent personnel would likely be. Thus, understaffing of permanent positions is a major concern for the DGMQ. While TERM NTE staff are important for filling the current gaps resulting from high turnover of FTE employees, the long-term stability and effectiveness of the DGMQ requires a steady FTE workforce.

There are likely multiple reasons for the dramatic split between permanent and nonpermanent staff. In addition to the funding issues described in the previous section, representatives of the DGMQ reported a range of challenges associated with recruiting and retaining permanent staff, including greater demands and consequent strain on human resource time (e.g., onboarding, badging, medical clearances) (Damon, 2022). The work required for contracting—including maintaining contracts and the administrative hurdles involved in filling other types of positions—is significant and time consuming. Furthermore, the training requirements and requisite oversight given to nonpermanent, temporary employees can cause inefficiency and increased demands on individual entities or the entire division. These requirements are incredibly challenging during emergency responses.

---

[12] Few of those unfunded positions are critical to the DGMQ sustainable infrastructure support for program and mission funds, so the DGMQ will align core programming dollars to funding these staffing needs.

Response Surge Staffing Challenges

Over the years, a continuing challenge for the DGMQ has been the need to staff surge responses with the right number of personnel, with the appropriate skill sets, in a timely manner. This challenge is underpinned by a host of issues (Roohi, 2022). For example, quickly hiring and onboarding new staff is difficult due to human resource constraints and challenging federal hiring procedures. During larger responses in particular—for example, emergencies such as the COVID-19 pandemic—there are competing staff needs of other CDC response components and task forces. Similar issues relate to non-CDC personnel—for example, Public Health Service surge staffing requires mission prioritization and approval from the U.S. Public Health Service Headquarters, given the substantial needs that also exist in other agencies.

When surge staff are identified, additional issues relate to the provision of national security clearance and badging requirements for physical access to restricted areas at U.S. ports, further impeding the speed of response capacity. Moreover, there are potential delays related to onboarding and administrative processes for arranging travel and medical clearance prior to domestic and international deployments. Skill set issues and training resource requirements can pose further barriers, especially when response needs are time sensitive. In the current and previous responses, the DGMQ onboarded a small number of CDC retirees on a temporary basis; however, this is not a sustainable solution due to the length of time involved in this process and the relatively small number of interested retirees. The DGMQ has also attempted to utilize nonfederal volunteer surge staff, but this gave rise to similar issues around security and medical clearance requirements, badging requirements, and access to IT systems.

Quarantine Station Staffing Challenges

Staffing of quarantine stations is also associated with a specific set of challenges. For instance, many tasks performed by quarantine station staff are largely administrative and do not require technical skills (such as medical training), while others—such as evaluating passengers for quarantinable diseases—require medical skills. In the past, the quarantine stations were staffed by well-trained public health administrators (i.e., quarantine officers). In recent years, however, the DGMQ has prioritized staffing quarantine stations with medical officers to facilitate screening needs. There may be opportunities to accomplish these screening needs by implementing technological solutions such as telemedicine (see Chapter 4) that could both reduce the workload on overburdened staff and minimize the need for positions requiring certain skill sets that may be more difficult to fill. In addition, medical professionals such as emergency medical technicians or nurse practitioners could be available on-site with doctors available remotely as needed.

Other challenges pertain to the operational hours and shift work at quarantine stations. Presently, many quarantine stations operate in a single daytime shift (i.e., 9:00 AM–5:00 PM) with varying degrees of after-hours coverage and on-call response. Based on experience during the response to the COVID-19 pandemic and other recent emergencies, a single shift does not adequately meet the necessary operational needs that are demanded. The arrival of passengers, cargo, and animals through designated U.S. ports of entry can occur at any time during a 24-hour day. This often requires staff members to work extended hours, to conduct public health consults remotely from home, or to return to the station during designated nonworking periods. This consistent occurrence during continuous high operational tempo inevitably leads to decreased morale, employee burnout, and increased turnover rates.

The Need for Competent Employees

The skills that workers need can change over the course of a few years (World Economic Forum, 2016). This is especially true for the DGMQ that operates in complex networks and relationships, needs significant technological advances and digital talent, works in a globally interconnected structure, and works as a regulator in the midst of the larger CDC that is almost entirely nonregulatory. Organizations in today's rapidly changing and complex environment need to "upskill" their workforce. Upskilling is a professional development strategy to augment the knowledge, skills, and competencies that help employees advance their careers and become more productive. It is a key tool to recruit, retain, and develop workers for organizational growth (Vroman and Danko, 2022). Some of the key skills recommended include collaboration, communication, creativity, critical thinking, cultural sensitivity, adaptation, transdisciplinary abilities, and ability to work across professions and organizations (Davies et al., 2011). Hiring and developing employees with pertinent skills is a key part of planning for its future workforce.

Challenges Related to Vacancy and Turnover Rates

As described, high vacancy and turnover rates across DGMQ staffing pose substantial challenges. Among the many reasons for vacancies and turnover are burnout, lack of adequate staff, and consequent overburdening of existing staff, especially increased overtime demands. Notably, early-mid career personnel—for example, GS-9 and GS-11 categories—tend to leave their positions at the DGMQ more frequently, which represents a loss of future leaders in the pipeline. Not only are many leaving the DGMQ, but they are increasingly leaving the CDC altogether—a significant challenge to be addressed, due to its consequences for both existing bench strength and the potential future of the DGMQ public health workforce.

The DGMQ staff have worked huge amounts of overtime hours to meet the needs and demands of recent major response efforts, which raises concerns of staff burnout and the DGMQ's ability to maintain mission-critical or regulatory work. Between 2019 and 2020, there was a drastic increase in the number of overtime hours worked, of 2,428 percent, which was aligned with COVID-19 spikes (Damon, 2022).[13] An initial very high peak of overtime work occurred in January 2020, reflecting the efforts to establish entry screening and support repatriation quarantine and isolation. Another peak occurred in July 2020. During this time, other staffing sources (e.g., U.S. Public Health Service Commissioned Corps Headquarters deployments) supported the DGMQ response, along with the CDC Emergency Operations Center (EOC) responders and deployers. An interagency agreement with the Department of Homeland Security Countering Weapons of Mass Destruction Office (CWMD) was also established to support screening, and other contract mechanisms were established for surge staffing. Although the steep increase in overtime hours worked moderated compared to the beginning of the pandemic, the number still remained higher than the baseline. Throughout late 2020 and into 2021, smaller peaks in overtime hours occurred with each successive wave of COVID-19 due to emerging variants of interest or concern in the United States.

At quarantine stations in particular, high turnover and vacancies made it difficult to conduct outbreak responses (Council of State and Territorial Epidemiologists, 2021). Overtime hours have seen an especially significant increase among more experienced workers—that is, those with higher GS levels (Damon, 2022).

The quarantine station network plays a critical role in the frontline protection of our borders from the introduction of communicable diseases. Excessive vacancies within the quarantine station network and the inability to retain skilled and experienced staff jeopardize the ability of the DGMQ to accomplish its core mission of protecting the United States from the introduction of communicable diseases. Thus, the appropriate staffing of authorized positions within the individual quarantine stations is a critical necessity that needs to remain a priority for the DGMQ.

---

[13] A caveat is that this percentage does not represent the additional efforts of certain staff types that are compensated differently (e.g., not eligible for overtime).

Potential Solutions to Workforce Challenges

The committee identified a range of potential solutions to the DGMQ's workforce challenges previously outlined. These include developing strategies to ensure adequate staffing, implementing changes to quarantine station operations, leveraging technology and telemedicine, and providing training opportunities. Among the primary needs is a standing "reserve force" of personnel that are able to be deployed at the outset of an emergency. In order to be ready when needed, this force would need to be in place before the emergency begins. Personnel need to be recruited, vetted by HR, and have received all necessary credentials so that the force is in place before an emergency occurs, saving precious time and effort in the response. Such a reserve corps would need to be composed of individuals that have critically needed skill sets to meet DGMQ emergency operational needs and who could immediately fill unoccupied temporary positions. These positions could be filled by federal employees, including from the CDC, or other contracted staff that are prepared to be deployed as soon as the need arises. The armed forces or HHS National Health Service Corps might serve as a model for innovative recruitment strategies; they support tuition and provide stipends for students in exchange for a commitment to serve for a specified period of time.

Developing Strategies to Ensure Adequate Staffing

- The DGMQ can explore a range of options to ensure adequate staffing, including the following: Explore the CRMD CDC PHI fellowship program[14] and the Public Health Associate Program[15] as a means of recruiting.
- Partner with local jurisdictions to hire or assign staff to work in the quarantine stations.
- Develop MOUs (Memoranda of Understanding) with other HHS agencies or the Public Health Service (PHS) to assign or detail their personnel to the quarantine stations.
- Develop MOUs with other federal agencies (e.g., Department of Homeland Security, Department of Transportation, Department of Defense) to assign or designate their personnel to work in the quarantine stations. The MOUs should better delineate the roles and responsibilities of the DGMQ versus its agency partners.
- Establish division-specific HR services to address challenges related

---

[14] More information on the CDC PHI fellowship program can be found at: https://phi-cdcfellows.org (accessed March 15, 2022).

[15] More information on the Public Health Associate Program can be found at: https://www.cdc.gov/phap/index.html (accessed March 15, 2022).

to routine HR processes to expedite training and clearance to on-board surges of staff.

Implementing Changes to Quarantine Station Operations

The DGMQ leadership has expressed the division's willingness to establish a goal that enables all quarantine stations to remain operational daily, utilizing two personnel shifts to provide 24-hour coverage. This change appears necessary and an appropriate common standard to implement across the network based on recent response requirements. However, the current high number of vacancies, which varies between quarantine stations, and the high number of TERM NTE positions will make this standard challenging—if not impossible—to meet for the entire network. Furthermore, if required, this will create more significant challenges to meet the demand of adding additional quarantine stations to the network.

A comprehensive plan needs to be developed to allocate the appropriate number of personnel required to fully operate two personnel shifts daily at each quarantine station and to conduct 24-hour operations during surges to DGMQ response requirements. This plan will need to focus on developing an increased number of permanent positions over the heavily reliant temporary positions; it should also include a thorough evaluation of the requirements to determine the requisite number of positions, competencies, job series, and grades needed at each station. Additionally, such a plan could also consider the use of available technologies that could reduce or eliminate some of the staff tasks and requirements currently being performed and minimize the need for extended hours and extra shifts. The development of a model prototype quarantine station could be beneficial. The design of a new maritime station—and perhaps additional air and/or land stations—could integrate personnel changes resulting from technology advances and collaboration with other federal organizations. Once new operating procedures and methods have been refined, the model could be scaled and used in other stations.

Leveraging Technology and Telemedicine

The DGMQ has an opportunity to also explore opportunities to leverage technology and telemedicine to alleviate the burden of responsibilities on its staff or potentially obviate the need for onsite medical officers. The COVID-19 pandemic has demonstrated the viability and value of telemedicine and digital support tools in preserving health care resources during an emergency response (Shen et al., 2021). For example, Mayo Clinic—the largest U.S. health care system—reported a 78 percent decrease in in-person health care visits from mid-March to mid-April 2020 and a 10,880 percent increase in video appointments during that same time frame (Marin, 2020). Now established in many countries, telemedicine platforms enable direct interactions between health care providers conducting consultations and their patients for health care visits. Moreover, teletechnology is available that can remotely collect data—such as blood pressure, heart rate, body temperature, recordings of the heart and lungs, and imaging of the ears, mouth, and skin—and transmit it to the health care provider in real time.

In briefings to the committee, quarantine authorities from other countries presented information about the implementation of various digital tools. These include electronic vaccination information and burner phones used to inform incoming passengers of public health risks and requirements. These tools offer benefits such as facilitating follow-up activities, avoiding issues associated with distribution of information in paper-based formats, and eliminating the need to manually enter information.[16] In planning to integrate telemedicine and digital technology, the DGMQ could consider

- contracting or utilizing a local private medical consultant or group;
- staffing a quarantine station with other medical professionals (e.g., nurses, physician assistants, nurse practitioners) with telemedicine backup within the DGMQ or elsewhere at the CDC;
- establishing a telemedicine agreement with a local clinic, hospital, or academic medical center; and
- establishing a telemedicine agreement with a national telemedicine service.

Providing Training Opportunities

To enhance workforce development opportunities for its staff and improve staff retention, strategies could be implemented to support training and education, as well as promoting staff wellness (Benenson, 2007). Once the staffing plan has been developed and appropriate skills and competencies have been identified, training and experiential learning needs can be determined for each job series.

The DGMQ already offers robust internal training opportunities for its staff that could be enhanced and expanded (Damon, 2022). For example, the DGMQ offers an internal Training and Transformational Leadership Upskilling Series, where it works to bring topics of broad interest into the division training series and strategizes to offer these opportunities to personnel at strategic times to increase attendance. The 2021 DGMQ Training Series was implemented to "(1) provide staff with requested trainings on priority topics, (2) offer opportunities and resources for DGMQ staff to add

---

[16] For further information on digital tools and technology in DGMQ, see Chapter 4.

knowledge and develop new skills for improving resiliency and institutional processes, and (3) create a more sustainable preparedness and response workforce infrastructure to address DGMQ's evolving needs in global migration and quarantine" (Damon, 2022). In 2021, the DGMQ Training Series had almost 1,000 attendees. The DGMQ's 2021 Transformational Leadership Upskilling Workshop—which had almost 500 attendees—was designed to develop future leaders and to invest in promoting leadership skills at all levels (Damon, 2022). It also contributes to building the DGMQ's public health workforce pipeline. Transformational leadership theory is used as a foundation to help staff become dynamic team members and leaders.

The CDC has developed a series of training programs aimed at advancing employee careers, reimaging organizational goals, and fostering employee well-being. CDC University, an internal training program, provides courses and pathways for enhanced competencies within an employee's job series or discipline. Courses are offered both in-person and virtually. CDC University's Compassion Institute was established with the goal of promoting compassion as a key component of its programs and activities in order to advance societal well-being through the organization. The DGMQ helped create and pilot CDC University's "Caring from the Inside Out" Training Initiative, which focuses on employee well-being, including sessions on mitigating stress and burnout and practicing self-care. Trained facilitators guide these 6-week sessions to provide participants with resources to improve work and home life (Damon, 2022).

In addition to the professional development trainings previously listed, the QBHSB provides robust routine and response-specific training to its staff. Upon joining the branch, staff received training plans with 20–40 operational courses tailored to their specific role. Courses usually have quizzes that must be completed to finish the course, and most courses must be repeated every 1–2 years to ensure staff are refreshed on content. The branch also creates partner training materials for station staff to use during their onsite trainings of port and public health partners. The branch also created and maintains a robust train-the-trainer program for CBP staff at the Federal Law Enforcement Training Center (FLETC) in Glynco, GA—where new CBP officers receive their basic training, including training in supporting CDC quarantine station operations. Through training a cadre of 10–20 FLETC trainers to deliver the CDC module 60+ times a year, the DGMQ empowers the CBP to partner in training and saves a significant amount of staff time and resources in traveling to the FLETC to deliver training. The CDC also augments CBP training at ports of entry (POE) through developing and delivering just-in-time trainings as needed on response operations (e.g., COVID-19 testing and vaccination requirements before boarding, COVID-19 public health risk assessments, etc.).

In addition to in-house training activities, the DGMQ could partner with academic institutions—including schools of public health and administration—to supplement and expand training activities. Partnering with schools of public health and administration could help to develop a pipeline of well-trained students that could fill positions within the division, including at the quarantine stations. Participation could be encouraged by providing potential incentives for graduates to work at the CDC, including loan repayment programs or scholarships. Students could also undertake experiential training while in school as interns or in other roles.

CULTURE

An organization's culture is defined by its system of collective beliefs, values, norms, behaviors, and artefacts (Cox et al., 2018). Culture represents an organization's "DNA" and helps to determine its actions and relationships. It is interwoven into the DGMQ's staffing issues and chronic underresourcing. Without an in-depth culture audit, the committee was limited in assessing this dimension of the DGMQ. However, there are a number of challenges that may be contributing to a culture at the DGMQ that limits its organizational capacity. These include structural constraints (e.g., inadequate financial and human resources), chronic vacancy rates, large amounts of overtime, diminished work-life balance, potential burnout and some industry relationships that may shape new norms and reflect a changing value system.

An organization's climate is different from its culture and describes the shared perception of people about an organization's policies, procedures, rewards, and personnel system. As such, the current difficulties in recruitment and retention may be critical climate issues and represent how others perceive the division. Other important culture considerations include ensuring that the DGMQ is a learning organization with an emphasis on continuous improvement and integration of knowledge; its ability to adapt, pivot, and be innovative; its commitment to diversity, equity, and inclusion; its levels of wellness and resilience; and its tolerance toward risk and transformational change.

The committee noted that the DGMQ recently instituted a Transformational Leadership training program with the Compassion Institute, designed to help staff become effective team members and dynamic leaders. The division has also established other internal training projects that are positive steps. However, more needs to be done. The DGMQ needs to invest further in leadership development and succession planning. Additional attention is needed in health, wellness, and resilience to address burnout, and work–life balance. The DGMQ needs to foster a supportive and diverse work environment to nurture a climate that maximizes its capacity to achieve the division's goals and to protect employees from experiencing any negative or long-term effects.

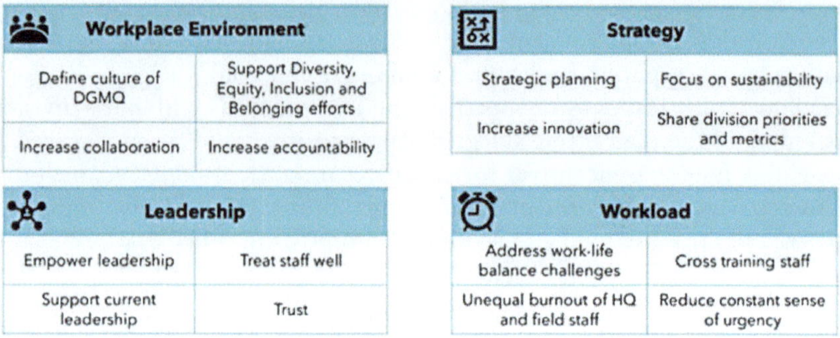

Workplace Environment	
Define culture of DGMQ	Support Diversity, Equity, Inclusion and Belonging efforts
Increase collaboration	Increase accountability

Strategy	
Strategic planning	Focus on sustainability
Increase innovation	Share division priorities and metrics

Leadership	
Empower leadership	Treat staff well
Support current leadership	Trust

Workload	
Address work-life balance challenges	Cross training staff
Unequal burnout of HQ and field staff	Reduce constant sense of urgency

FIGURE 2-4 Focus areas for DGMQ culture.
SOURCE: Damon, 2022, slide 97.

The DGMQ is currently exploring opportunities to support and enhance its workforce culture, with a focus on four key areas: workplace environment, strategy, leadership, and workload (see Figure 2-4) (Damon, 2022). Within the domain of workplace environment, efforts are focused on (1) crystallizing and defining the culture of the DGMQ; (2) supporting diversity, equity, inclusion, and belonging efforts; (3) fostering greater collaboration; and (4) increasing accountability. Strategy efforts involve strategic planning, increasing innovation, focusing on sustainability, and sharing the division's priorities and metrics. Efforts to enhance leadership include empowering and supporting leadership, treating staff well, and building trust. In the focus area of addressing workload, opportunities include (1) addressing work-life balance challenges, (2) exploring ways to reduce the unequal burnout of headquarters and field staff, (3) cross-training staff, and (4) reducing the constant sense of urgency.

CONCLUSIONS AND RECOMMENDATIONS

The current level of funding and personnel for the Quarantine Station Program of the DGMQ is inadequate and is preventing the organization from effectively and efficiently carrying out its many responsibilities and activities. The continuous challenge of emergencies and pandemics over the last decade have stretched the DGMQ's capacity and ability to respond to global disease threats.

The committee's assessment of the agency's organizational capacity finds that it is designed to operate in a past era—before the last decade's unprecedented and profound health events. The DGMQ has had to leap from crisis to crisis by trying to use surge funds, temporary workers, and contract workers to meet these profound challenges. Unfortunately, operating in persistent emergency mode with inadequate staff and other resources has become the norm. Even after the COVID-19 pandemic has subsided, it is highly unlikely that the organization will ever return to "normal." New outbreaks and emergencies are the new normal, and the surge requirements seen over the last decade are not an aberration. Thus, now is an inflection point for the DGMQ that calls into question how it works, what it works on, with whom it works, when it works, and if it will ever have sufficient resources and a modern infrastructure to carry out its mandate and meet present and future public health challenges. The status quo is not an acceptable strategy.

The committee acknowledges that the DGMQ has implemented a number of successful changes and actions since the report on the agency 15 years ago (Institute of Medicine, 2006). The addition of quarantine stations and increased capacity for testing and tracing mark needed progress. Although mostly successful in the past, however, the DGMQ needs to confront and change many of its legacy programs, systems, and behaviors as it faces a more uncertain and complex future. Changing trends in global travel have vastly outpaced institutional changes within the DGMQ. The division's current structure, including its finances and staffing, is drastically underprepared to meet demands of the modern global context. It is clear that the current limitations on funding and personnel are inadequate for the DGMQ's quarantine stations to effectively carry out their responsibilities and mission.

There is an opportunity to redesign quarantine stations, adopting new technologies and innovations (digital and diagnostic platforms), altering workload and operational hours, incorporating telehealth, working smarter, and creating a network of modern quarantine stations for the future. The organization needs a contemporary personnel plan and culture audit that resolves key issues such as high vacancy rates, excessive overtime work, a preponderance of temporary and contract employees, burnout, turnover (especially in younger employees who represent the leaders of the future), skills and competencies compatible with the changing needs of their jobs, an innovative and exciting recruiting plan, and tools and programs to ensure resiliency. The committee notes that standalone organizations—including entities with a "Center" designation—are better able to manage finances and personnel in addition to allowing for more senior positions to facilitate recruitment, retention, and professional advancement opportunities.

The committee's findings and conclusions are not a reflection of the many outstanding people of the DGMQ, but rather a reflection of its difficult times and how the organization needs to realign itself to meet contemporary needs and technological advances. In today's context, any organization that cannot rethink and reimage is unlikely to be successful.

Conclusions

Conclusion 2-1: Due to its critical role in ensuring national health security, the DGMQ may benefit from a more prominent position in the CDC's organizational structure.

Conclusion 2-2: The DGMQ has a broad range of responsibilities that extend beyond its primary scope, such as the distribution of drugs.

Conclusion 2-3: Data management systems to track travelers could facilitate disease detection, surveillance, and contact tracing.

Conclusion 2-4: Additional engagement of aviation and maritime industries could assist in communicable disease control.

Conclusion 2-5: Current base funding is not commensurate with current DGMQ responsibilities. Cycles of surge funding do not support a sustainable, proactive system that is ready to be deployed as soon as a public health emergency is identified. Recalibration of the DGMQ's baseline funding would help the division meet the challenges of today's expansive border health landscape and heightened threats of novel infectious disease outbreaks, thus enabling the DGMQ to meet its growing responsibilities and to be better prepared for a complex, uncertain, and demanding future.

Conclusion 2-6: A pandemic fund that explicitly mentions the DGMQ as a recipient could allow the DGMQ to nimbly access funds during crises while awaiting legislative appropriation. Emergency/pandemic funds that are readily accessible and of sufficient amounts are needed to enable the DGMQ to respond to the next emergency more quickly and effectively than its current capability.

Conclusion 2-7: Identifying pathogens for prioritization would be valuable to focus efforts and response possibilities. The DGMQ could consider appropriate prioritization schematics in generating responses and targeting resources.[17]

Conclusion 2-8: The DGMQ is currently not appropriately staffed and therefore cannot effectively discharge its responsibilities and ac-

---

[17] In 2021, a workshop was held to prioritize pathogens in the U.S.–Mexico border region that are of concern to U.S. federal and state partners (see https://www.cdc.gov/usmexicohealth/pdf/onehealth-southernus-508.pdf). Conducting further pathogen prioritization relevant to all ports of entry would be beneficial.

complish its mission. Staff currently work extended hours and take on extra shifts, leading to staff burnout and turnover.

Conclusion 2-9: *The DGMQ's heavy reliance on nonpermanent staff, such as fellows and contractors, is an inefficient way to operate and to accomplish its range of critical activities. This reliance on nonpermanent staff is likely to affect the functioning of the division, its workplace culture, and the morale of the permanent staff.*

Conclusion 2-10: *The availability of modern technologies could influence the requisite skill sets of personnel assigned to quarantine stations. While medical consultation is clearly needed for the quarantine stations to fulfill their responsibilities, options that do not rely on on-site medical officers to reduce the work burden may be viable. Establishing a telemedicine agreement with national telemedicine service*

Conclusion 2-11: *If the DGMQ gained designation as a Center, it would be eligible to gain more support staff and be eligible for higher-level grades and positions which would help with staff retention. It would also result in more readily available funding.*

Recommendations

Recommendation 2-1: The U.S. Department of Health and Human Services (HHS), especially including the Centers for Disease Control and Prevention (CDC), should ensure that the Division of Global Migration and Quarantine (DGMQ) has the necessary financial and personnel resources, an effective organizational structure, and optimal infrastructure to effectively meet its responsibilities, execute its growing volume of work, and achieve its mission.

To implement this recommendation, the DGMQ needs to specifically act and resolve the following issues:
A. Organizational restructuring
 1. Strong consideration should be given to restructuring the DGMQ to become a standalone unit with a direct reporting line to the CDC director.
B. Finances
 1. HHS should make a special agreement with the DGMQ to enable the DGMQ to utilize readily accessible funding in future emergencies. The process of acquiring and utilizing surge funds should be streamlined to facilitate greater flex-

ibility during both their acquisition and during the drawdown period post-emergency.
   2. The CDC should explore, along with the administration and Congress, the development of a user fee program to ensure that the division has a consistent and dependable source of revenue to cover the costs of operating the quarantine stations.
C. Workforce
   1. The DGMQ should develop and implement a comprehensive and contemporary personnel plan to address multiple issues of recruitment, retention, skills development, vacancy rates, burnout, and excessive reliance on contract and temporary staff. This plan should also include a commitment to diversity, equity, and inclusion, and to critical training needs and upskilling to prepare staff to successfully work in a dynamic, rapidly changing, and demanding environment and to stay abreast of evolving technologies. The plan should address the need for all quarantine stations to operate on a two-shift standard.
   2. The DGMQ should develop and launch innovative strategies to support its critical recruitment needs.
      a. The organization should work with academic entities, such as universities and schools of public health, medicine, and law to develop a pipeline of future employees. Creative incentives and a streamlined human resources (HR) process should be used to facilitate the recruitment of graduates.
      b. The DGMQ should design, develop, and implement a "Ready Reserve Corps": a well-trained, experienced, and agile group of personnel with essential competencies who are preapproved and cleared, and thus could be immediately available to rapidly meet personnel needs of the organization during emergencies. This group should be paid a stipend to serve, be on standby status, and engage in training and practice exercises.
   3. DGMQ should leverage opportunities presented through the CDC director's diversity, equity, and inclusion initiatives while undergoing the division's workforce study.
D. Culture
   The DGMQ should assess its organizational culture and climate in association with the personnel and development plan to ensure that the division's values positively support its mission. This assessment should include a focus on diversity, equity, and inclusion. Corrective actions should be initiated if findings suggest that an adjustment is needed.

Recommendation 2-2: The Division of Global Migration and Quarantine (DGMQ) should create an effective and innovative quarantine-station model that matches the expanding and changing needs of a global, mobile world and augments its work in a progressively challenging infectious disease environment.

To achieve this recommendation, the DGMQ needs to implement these specific steps:

A. Develop criteria to determine whether a quarantine station should be added, deleted, or upgraded, and adjust the current number of stations accordingly. If a new station is deemed necessary, conduct a business plan during preplanning to determine (1) the optimal number of staff to support a two-shift standard, (2) requisite staff competencies, (3) necessary support staff, and (4) capacity for routine round-the-clock coverage during emergencies if needed. If a new station is deemed necessary, conduct a business plan during preplanning to (5) determine whether the new site could have multiple uses and (6) identify potential partners that the new site could engage between and during emergencies. Finally, (7) adopt appropriate advanced technology including telemedicine options.

B. The maritime unit should be permanently housed within the DGMQ so that it can address the unique needs of the cruise industry and maritime-traveling public to enhance collaboration and disease control activities in maritime settings. The maritime quarantine station should have transparent operations and strong partnerships with regulated parties and other relevant entities.

C. Develop a more robust program for preclearance of passengers, immigrants, and animals, including collaborative actions with other pertinent agencies and organizations. The emphasis would be on upstream locations outside of the United States to ease workload at entry sites.

D. Redesign post-entry follow-ups in partnership with local and state agencies, and other federal agencies, in which resources and responsibilities are better shared and modern technology is used for communications, tracking, and surveillance.

REFERENCES

Alvarado-Ramy, F. 2022. *Quarantine and Border Health Services Branch: CDC, DGMQ*. Presentation to the National Academies of Sciences, Engineering, and Medicine Committee on Analysis to Enhance the Effectiveness of the Federal Quarantine Station Network.

Benenson, G. 2007. *CDC's quarantine branch: Building partnerships and enhancing workforce development*. Paper presented at 135st APHA Annual Meeting and Exposition.

Brown, C., F. Alvarado-Ramy, and A. Klevos. 2021. *To screen or not to screen? There's more to border health than interventions at our borders*: CDC. Presentation to the National Academies of Sciences, Engineering, and Medicine Committee on Analysis to Enhance the Effectiveness of the Federal Quarantine Station Network.

Buigut, J., and B. A. Maskery. 2021. *CDC's Division of Global Migration and Quarantine: National Academy of Sciences DGMQ overview and COVID-19 regulatory activities*: CDC. Presentation to the National Academies of Sciences, Engineering, and Medicine Committee on Analysis to Enhance the Effectiveness of the Federal Quarantine Station Network.

CDC (Centers for Disease Control and Prevention). 2016. *Division and office overviews*. National Center for Emerging and Zoonotic Infectious Diseases (NCEZID). https://www.cdc.gov/ncezid/who-we-are/ncezid-divisions/index.html (accessed May 3, 2022).

CDC. 2019a. *How CDC's quarantine stations welcome new arrivals to the United States and protect the health of U.S. communities*. Atlanta, Georgia: Centers for Disease Control and Prevention. https://www.cdc.gov/ncezid/dgmq/feature-stories/quarantine-stations-arrivals.html (accessed February 18, 2022).

CDC. 2019b. *About the Vessel Sanitation Program*. https://www.cdc.gov/nceh/vsp/desc/about-vsp.htm (accessed April 27, 2022).

CDC. 2021a. *Laws and regulations*. Division of Global Migration and Quarantine (DGMQ). https://www.cdc.gov/ncezid/dgmq/laws-and-regulations.html (accessed May 18, 2022).

CDC. 2021b. *Emergency response*. Division of Global Migration and Quarantine (DGMQ). https://www.cdc.gov/ncezid/dgmq/emergency-response.html (accessed February 18, 2022).

CDC. 2021c. *Quarantine and border health services*. Division of Global Migration and Quarantine (DGMQ). https://www.cdc.gov/ncezid/dgmq/focus-areas/quarantine.html (accessed February 28, 2022).

CDC. 2021d. *Who we are*. Division of Global Migration and Quarantine (DGMQ). https://www.cdc.gov/ncezid/dgmq/who-we-are.html (accessed February 25, 2022).

CDC. 2022. *U.S. quarantine stations*. https://www.cdc.gov/quarantine/quarantine-stations-us.html (accessed February 16, 2022).

Cetron, M. 2021. *DGMQ's evolution since the 2006 NASEM report: Quarantine stations at ports of entry: Protecting the public's health*: CDC. Presentation to the National Academies of Sciences, Engineering, and Medicine Committee on Analysis to Enhance the Effectiveness of the Federal Quarantine Station Network.

Cohen, N. J., C. M. Brown, F. Alvarado-Ramy, H. Bair-Brake, G. A. Benenson, T. H. Chen, A. J. Demma, N. K. Holton, K. S. Kohl, A. W. Lee, D. McAdam, N. Pesik, S. Roohi, C. L. Smith, S. H. Waterman, and M. S. Cetron. 2016. Travel and border health measures to prevent the international spread of ebola. *MMWR: Morbidity and Mortality Weekly Report* 65(3):57-67.

Council of State and Territorial Epidemiologists. 2021. *Evaluation of jurisdictional & federal public health responses to past & current outbreaks & implementation of CSTE protocol for health department notification to CDC quarantine stations of infectious persons with recent travel*. Atlanta, Georgia: U.S. Council of State and Territorial Epidemiologists.

Cox, K., S. Jolly, S. Van Der Staaij, and C. Van Stolk. 2018. *Understanding the drivers of organisational capacity*. Santa Monica, California: RAND Corporation. https://doi.org/10.7249/RR2189.

Damon, J. 2022. *Review of budget and staffing—DGMQ funding, staffing, and turnover data 2019–2021*: CDC. Presentation to the National Academies of Sciences, Engineering, and Medicine Committee on Analysis to Enhance the Effectiveness of the Federal Quarantine Station Network.

Davies, A., D. Fidler, and M. Gorbis. 2011. *Future work skills 2020*. Palo Alto, California: Institute for the Future.

Department of Homeland Security. 2022. *DHS responds: Coronavirus (COVID-19)*. https://www.dhs.gov/coronavirus (accessed May 2, 2022).

Dollard, P., I. Griffin, A. Berro, N. J. Cohen, K. Singler, Y. Haber, C. de la Motte Hurst, A. Stolp, S. Atti, L. Hausman, C. E. Shockey, S. Roohi, C. M. Brown, L. D. Rotz, M. S. Cetron, CDC COVID-19 Port of Entry Team, and F. Alvarado-Ramy. 2020. Risk assessment and management of COVID-19 among travelers arriving at designated U.S. airports, January 17–September 13, 2020. *MMWR: Morbidity and Mortality Weekly Report* 69(45):1681-1685. http://dx.doi.org/10.15585/mmwr.mm6945a4.

FDA (U.S. Food and Drug Administration). 2022. *FDA user fee programs*. https://www.fda.gov/industry/fda-user-fee-programs (accessed March 16, 2022).

Hoffman, S. J., and M. J. P. Poirier. 2022. *The law, epidemiology and politics of COVID-19 national border closures: Global Strategy Lab*. Presentation to the National Academies of Sciences, Engineering, and Medicine Committee on Analysis to Enhance the Effectiveness of the Federal Quarantine Station Network.

Institute of Medicine. 2006. *Quarantine stations at ports of entry: Protecting the public's health*. Washington, DC: The National Academies Press.

Marin, A. 2020. Telemedicine takes center stage in the era of COVID-19. *Science* November 6.

Roohi, S. 2022. *Role of global migration task force (GMTF) in CDC Incident Management Structure (IMS): U.S. Centers for Disease Control and Prevention, Division of Global Migration and Quarantine*. Presentation to the National Academies of Sciences, Engineering, and Medicine Committee on Analysis to Enhance the Effectiveness of the Federal Quarantine Station Network.

Rosenthal, P. J., and K. R. Tan. 2019. Expanded availability of intravenous artesunate for the treatment of severe malaria in the United States. *The American Journal of Tropical Medicine and Hygiene* 100(6):1295-1296. https://doi.org/10.4269/ajtmh.19-0230.

Shen, Y. T., L. Chen, W. W. Yue, and H. X. Xu. 2021. Digital technology-based telemedicine for the COVID-19 pandemic. *Frontiers in Medicine* 8:646506. https://doi.org/10.3389/fmed.2021.646506.

Tardivel, K. M. D. 2022. *Maritime Unit: CDC*. Presentation to the National Academies of Sciences, Engineering, and Medicine Committee on Analysis to Enhance the Effectiveness of the Federal Quarantine Station Network.

Vroman, S. R., and T. Danko. 2022. How to build a successful upskilling program. *Harvard Business Review* January 18. https://hbr.org/2022/01/how-to-build-a-successful-upskilling-program (accessed May 18, 2022).

Walls, T. M. 2021. Federal quarantine: The issue with limited CDC presence at ports of entry. *Journal of Biosecurity, Biosafety and Biodefense Law* 12(1):175-191. https://doi.org/10.1515/jbbbl-2021-2009.

World Economic Forum. 2016. *The future of jobs: Employment, skills, and workforce strategy for the fourth industrial revolution*. Geneva, Switzerland: World Economic Forum.

3

Disease Control and Response Efforts

The core function of the Division of Global Migration and Quarantine (DGMQ) and its network of quarantine stations is the control of communicable human disease. Infectious disease threats are extremely varied in terms of virulence, severity, transmission potential, epidemic potential, and potential public health consequences. Disease control tools used by the DGMQ have common themes, but also are tailored to the specific threats based on these variables. Over the past two decades, the pace and variance of infectious disease threats to the United States have been accelerating at an alarming rate. This likely reflects a range of factors including greater ease of travel, increasing speed and range of international travel, escalating emergence of novel pathogens, and improved communication and diagnostic tools.

THE DGMQ'S ROLES AND RESPONSIBILITIES IN COMMUNICABLE DISEASE CONTROL

The DGMQ has a range of domestic and international roles in its responsibility for controlling the spread of communicable diseases at both international air and maritime ports of entry and at land-border crossings.[1] The DGMQ's day-to-day responsibilities focus on responding to travelers, animals, human remains, and products that may have specific communicable diseases of public health concern upon their entry to the United

---

[1] More information about the DGMQ's roles and responsibilities is available from https://www.cdc.gov/ncezid/dgmq/how-we-serve.html (accessed March 15, 2022).

States by air, sea, or land.² When major communicable disease threats emerge within the United States or abroad—such as outbreaks of potential or definite pandemic potential—the DGMQ can leverage its existing partnerships and expand its ordinary operations and activities as part of the emergency response to help prevent the introduction and spread of disease into the United States or across its borders. In recent decades, the DGMQ has supported infection control efforts for a broad range of communicable diseases, such as tuberculosis (TB)—including both multidrug-resistant tuberculosis (MDR-TB) and extensively drug-resistant TB (XDR-TB)—Ebola virus disease, Zika virus disease, Lassa fever, measles, chikungunya virus disease, monkeypox, rabies, extensively drug-resistant typhoid, the 2009 H1N1 influenza pandemic, Middle East respiratory syndrome (MERS)-CoV, SARS-CoV-1 (the virus that causes severe acute respiratory syndrome [SARS]), SARS-CoV-2 (the virus that causes COVID-19), and cholera.

The DGMQ's Day-to-Day Activities

The DGMQ's day-to-day responsibilities generally pertain to individual travelers and are primarily aimed at responding to communicable diseases of public health concern in arriving travelers, as well as importations that pose a potential public health threat. For individual travelers, the DGMQ's suite of infectious disease control tools includes public health travel restrictions—specifically the Do Not Board (DNB) list and the Public Health Lookout—and contact investigations, and issuance of public health orders for quarantine, isolation, or conditional release when necessary. Though the DGMQ's overall mission encompasses many areas of prevention, including travel health advice and vaccine recommendations, this section will focus on disease control measures.

Air Travel Responsibilities

Airlines and U.S. Customs and Border Protection (CBP) also play critical roles in detecting and responding to ill travelers and containing the spread of communicable diseases. These activities are maintained between outbreak or pandemic periods and may be scaled up during a global pandemic. Staff at quarantine stations may be notified of potentially ill travelers before, during, or after travel. When quarantine station staff are notified of an ill traveler, they communicate with quarantine medical officers, who guide staff on the actions necessary to appropriately mitigate communicable diseases risks. The appropriate steps to mitigate this risk will depend on

---

² This text was modified after release of the report to the study sponsor to correctly represent the division's responsibilities.

whether the CDC is notified before, during, or after travel. Quarantine station staff enter the information regarding the ill traveler(s) and any actions taken into the secure Quarantine Activity Reporting System (QARS).

For passengers identified before travel or during travel, health departments may ask to have travelers added to the DNB list and the Public Health Lookout if they meet established criteria—that is, if they are reasonably believed to be infectious with or at risk of becoming infectious with a communicable disease of public health importance that poses a risk to the traveling public and are at risk for travel, or are not adherent to public health recommendations, or are unaware of their diagnosis. More information is provided in the Travel Restrictions section, which follows.

Ill (or dead) travelers identified during travel can include passengers or crew identified while on board conveyances or travelers identified at transportation hubs by federal and nonfederal partners. If an air passenger is observed with signs of illness that meet the Centers for Disease Control and Prevention's (CDC's) regulatory definition, or a death occurs on board, the pilot of the aircraft must report the situation to the CDC quarantine station with jurisdiction for the arrival airport.[3] Before the aircraft lands, the pilot must provide details such as aircraft identification, the departure airport, the destination airport, estimated time of arrival, number of persons on board the aircraft, number of suspected case(s) on board, and the nature of the public health risk if it is known. If the CBP or other partners identify an ill traveler upon arrival, they may also notify the quarantine station with jurisdiction. The CDC provides CBP officers and other airport partners, including emergency medical services, with job aids (i.e., "RING" cards that remind CBP officers to Recognize, Isolate, Notify, and Give support) to support this function. This partnership is especially important at airports where the DGMQ does not have staff on site.

The Quarantine and Border Health Services Branch (QBHSB) also works closely with CBP personnel at designated foreign airports where travelers are inspected by the CBP prior to boarding U.S.-bound flights (i.e., preclearance ports of entry) to ensure consistent application of CDC regulatory requirements for these travelers and any CDC-regulated items they may attempt to import. This work is performed remotely and primarily consists of periodic outreach and the provision of job aids.

Quarantine stations may also receive reports, typically from health departments, for travelers who were diagnosed with communicable diseases after travel. Quarantine station staff will work with quarantine medical officers to determine whether a contact investigation should be initiated.

---

[3] More information about the CDC's protocol for reporting onboard deaths and illnesses is available from https://www.cdc.gov/quarantine/air/reporting-deaths-illness/guidance-reporting-onboard-deaths-illnesses.html (accessed February 22, 2022).

More information on the Electronic Passenger Reporting System used for contact investigations is reported in a separate section, which follows.[4] In 2019, the Council of State and Territorial Epidemiologists (CSTE), with support from the CDC, evaluated reports to the DGMQ of infectious travelers in order to assess processes that state and local epidemiologists use to report ill travelers with diseases of public health concern to the QBHSB. The CSTE identified areas for improvement for both state and territorial epidemiologists and the CDC's DGMQ (Council of State and Territorial Epidemiologists, 2020).

The DGMQ also supports efforts with partners to develop Communicable Disease Response Plans (CDRPs), which provide the basis for a multisector and multistate response to a public health disaster/emergency at ports of entry. This is accomplished through federal regulatory enforcement at ports of entry and by supporting local, state, and tribal public health agencies during domestic travel communicable disease responses, as requested, to prevent the introduction, transmission, or spread of communicable diseases.

Federal Public Health Travel Restrictions

Two public health tools for communicable disease control used by federal authorities are the DNB list and the Public Health Lookout.[5] These tools—managed jointly by the U.S. Department of Homeland Security (DHS) and the CDC—were established in 2007. The DNB list prevents individuals known or suspected to have a communicable disease that poses a public health threat from being issued a boarding pass for any commercial airplane traveling into, within, or out of the United States. Additionally, to facilitate public health notification, these individuals are also issued a Public Health Lookout to allow them to be identified if they seek entry to the United States at an airport, land, or sea port of entry.[6]

In cases where an individual who poses a public health risk intends to travel, local and state public health authorities can request assistance from the CDC to ensure that the individual does not travel while still infectious.[7] Individuals may be placed on the DNB list and issued a Lookout if they are

---

[4] See Protecting Travelers' Health from Airport to Community: Investigating Contagious Diseases on Flights | Quarantine | CDC https://www.cdc.gov/quarantine/contact-investigation.html (accessed April 3, 2022).

[5] More information about these travel restriction tools is available from https://www.cdc.gov/quarantine/travel-restrictions.html (accessed March 15, 2022).

[6] See https://www.federalregister.gov/documents/2015/03/27/2015-07118/criteria-for-requesting-federal-travel-restrictions-for-public-health-purposes-including-for-viral (accessed May 21, 2022).

[7] See https://www.cdc.gov/quarantine/travel-restrictions.html (accessed May 21, 2022).

"known or believed to be infectious with, or at risk for, a serious contagious disease that poses a public health threat to others during travel" and meet at least one of the following three criteria: (1) the individual is not aware of the diagnosis or not following public health recommendations, (2) the individual is likely to travel on a commercial flight involving the United States or travel internationally by any means, or (3) a travel restriction needs to be issued to respond to a public health outbreak or to help enforce a public health order (CDC, 2022f). The CDC reviews the records of all individuals subject to these restrictions every 2 weeks to assess their eligibility for removal of restrictions. After public health authorities determine that an individual is no longer infectious or at risk of becoming infectious, the person's information is removed from both tools (CDC, 2022f).

During the COVID-19 pandemic, these federal public health tools have been used to restrict travel by individuals with COVID-19 and their close contacts who are recommended to quarantine. These authorities can also be utilized to restrict travel by individuals with other suspected or confirmed infectious diseases that could threaten public health during travel. Before the COVID-19 pandemic, most uses of federal public health travel restrictions were for people with infectious TB; however, the tools have also been used for measles, MERS, Ebola virus disease, and Lassa fever.[8]

When an individual on the Public Health Lookout enters the United States, the CDC is notified by CBP officers at the point of entry; a public health evaluation is then performed prior to the individual's release (DeSisto et al., 2015). The CDC's Quarantine Public Health Officers are responsible for (1) notifying the relevant local and state public health authorities that an individual on the Public Health Lookout has been identified and (2) working with local and state authorities to conduct the appropriate public health interventions, including isolation, coordinated treatment referral, and compliance with any established federal and state legal measures (CDC, 2022f; DeSisto et al., 2015).

The DNB and Lookout lists have been most commonly used for people with suspected or confirmed infectious TB, including MDR-TB. TB is a curable, preventable, but potentially serious infectious disease that is not highly transmissible. However, an individual with active (i.e., infectious) pulmonary TB can transmit the disease during periods of prolonged close contact, such as air travel (Martinez et al., 2010). Despite federally mandated overseas TB screening for immigrants and refugees, the CDC reports that there are about 125 active TB cases per year among arriving travelers including visitors, students, and temporary workers (Kim et al., 2012). The escalating rates of MDR-TB and XDR-TB warrant major concerns regard-

---

[8] See https://www.cdc.gov/quarantine/travel-restrictions.html (accessed May 21, 2022).

ing transmission into the United States at both air and land-border points of entry (Salzer et al., 2016).

Health screenings also occur at quarantine stations to assess passengers for illness who may not be on a DNB or Public Health Lookout. This form of surveillance can vary depending on context, such the event of a public health emergency. During the West Africa Ebola outbreak of 2014–2016, passengers from affected countries went through exit screening prior to leaving the country.[9] This included temperature checks, answering health questions, and visual assessment for illness. Those who arrived in the United States were subject to entry screening. Passengers who had traveled through Guinea, Sierra Leone, or Liberia underwent screenings that included answering questions about potential risk, temperature checks, and observation for other Ebola symptoms. Staff at all U.S. international airports were trained to respond to any reports of ill travelers (CDC and DHS, 2014).[10] During the COVID-19 pandemic, regulations surrounding screenings changed throughout the course of the pandemic. In February 2020, all incoming flights from China were directed to 11 U.S. airports. At these airports, "[i]ncoming passengers [were] screened for fever, cough, and shortness of breath. Any travelers with signs or symptoms of illness receive[d] a more comprehensive public health assessment" (Jernigan, 2020). As of December 6, 2021, prior to boarding a flight bound for the United States, international travelers must show either (1) documentation of a recent negative COVID-19 test or (2) documentation of recent recovery from COVID-19 infection with a physician's note clearing the passenger for travel (U.S. Department of State, 2022).

The challenge of passenger screening and enacting public health measures is highlighted by the increase in the number of travelers to the United States over the past several years. The number of international arrivals in U.S. airports increased from about 80 million in 2006 to about 120 million in 2019. These numbers dropped to ~30 million in 2020 and 20 million in 2021 (Maskery, 2022). The volume of travelers arriving via land borders does not demonstrate as significant a change, but still represents a large population that requires screening. International land border arrivals have gone from a high of nearly 300 million in 2006 to approximately 210 million in 2011. Numbers of arrivals ranged from 210 to 250 million between 2011 and 2019. This number dropped to 115 million in 2020, and rose only slightly to 130 million in 2021 as a result of restricted travel due to the COVID-19 pandemic (Maskery, 2022). The COVID-19 pandemic also resulted in a drastic increase in the number of illnesses detected in airports that warranted

---

[9] This text was modified after release of the report to the study sponsor to clarify which departing passengers were screened.

[10] This text was modified after release of the report to the study sponsor to specify which international airports had staff trained to respond to ill travelers.

responses. From 2016–2019, annual responses ranged from 1,300 to 1,500 responses before, during, or after travel. This number soared to over 35,000 in 2020, and to near 90,000 in 2021 (CDC, 2022f; Maskery, 2022).

Contact Investigations

Contact investigations are another tool used by the CDC and DGMQ to protect the health of individuals who have been exposed to an infectious disease during air travel and to prevent the forward spread of that disease in communities.[11] Historically, most flight contact investigations are conducted by the CDC in close coordination with state and local public health authorities for cases of infectious TB, measles, rubella, pertussis, meningococcal disease, and more recently for COVID-19. The CDC typically notifies state, tribal, local, and territorial (STLT) authorities about exposed persons in their jurisdictions and health departments then notify identified persons of their exposures and put in place appropriate disease control plans, including provision of post-exposure prophylaxis or vaccine when indicated.

A contact investigation is typically triggered after the CDC is notified by state or local public health authorities that an air traveler (i.e., the index patient) has sought treatment at a medical facility and has been diagnosed with a specific infectious disease, which can happen up to days or weeks after travel. In other situations, the CDC may be notified about an ill traveler who is currently on a plane, or has recently landed. The CDC is responsible for coordinating contact investigations on domestic flights, arriving international flights, land-border crossings, and cruises that were taken by the index patient.[12] Quarantine public health officers in consultation with the Quarantine Medical Officer evaluate whether the index patient was contagious during the flight and may have potentially exposed passengers seated nearby (i.e., contacts).[13] The CDC then requests the flight manifest[14] for those contacts and shares the passengers' information with the relevant state, local, or international public health authorities, who in turn try to locate the passengers to inform them about their potential exposure and recommended actions.

---

[11] More information about CDC contact investigations is available from https://www.cdc.gov/quarantine/contact-investigation.html (accessed March 15, 2022).

[12] This text was modified to correct the characterization of CDC's responsibilities for contact investigations.

[13] This text was modified after release of the report to the study sponsor to correctly describe who conducts the evaluations.

[14] The CDC protects passenger privacy and does not release any information about the index patient or the contacts beyond public health staff working on the investigation. This information is protected and its access is strictly limited to public health use (https://www.cdc.gov/quarantine/contact-investigation.html, accessed May 21, 2022).

Isolation and Quarantine

In relatively rare instances, the federal government exercises its legal authorities[15] to implement isolation and quarantine to help prevent the public's exposure to an individual who has or may have specific infectious diseases of great public health risk (CDC, 2021c). Isolation and quarantine functions differ, in that isolation separates individuals who are sick with a designated infectious disease of consequence from individuals who are not sick. The quarantine function separates and restricts the movement of people who were exposed to an infectious disease, in order to observe (or monitor) them to see if they become sick and to prevent them from exposing others during the period of time that they are potentially infectious.

An executive order of the president authorizes federal isolation and quarantine for a specific set of infectious diseases; this list can also be revised by the president through executive order. Currently, isolation and quarantine are federally authorized for cholera, diphtheria, infectious tuberculosis, plague, smallpox, yellow fever, viral hemorrhagic fevers, severe acute respiratory syndromes, novel influenza strains with pandemic potential, and measles.

The U.S. Department of Health and Human Services (HHS) has delegated the federal authority[16] to carry out isolation and quarantine functions to the CDC. If an individual has a suspected or confirmed case of one of the designated infectious diseases, the CDC can issue a federal isolation or quarantine order. An individual may be conditionally released from quarantine subject to compliance with medical monitoring and surveillance. Breaking a federal quarantine order is punishable by fines and imprisonment. In most scenarios, these orders are enforced with support from partners, such as federal, state, tribal, and/or local public health authorities; law enforcement officers; U.S. CBP officers; and U.S. Coast Guard officers.

Despite these authorities, individual federal isolation and quarantine powers are rarely used in practice and have been used even less frequently at large scale. There is generally heavy reliance on state and local health authorities to issue orders for isolation and quarantine. State and local officials usually have policies, procedures, staff, and structure in place to enforce these orders. Across the DGMQ's network of quarantine stations, infectious TB was the most frequently occurring infectious disease for

---

[15] The authority for isolation and quarantine derives from the Commerce Clause of the U.S. Constitution. Under section 361 of the Public Health Service Act (42 U.S. Code §264), the U.S. secretary of Health and Human Services is authorized to take measures to prevent the entry and spread of communicable diseases from foreign countries into the United States and between states. Isolation and quarantine also are considered "police power" functions that are derived from the state's right to take action affecting individuals for the benefit of society.

[16] Under 42 Code of Federal Regulations parts 70 and 71, the CDC is authorized to detain, medically examine, and release persons arriving into the United States and traveling between states who are suspected of carrying these communicable diseases.

which federal individual isolation was authorized between 2007 and 2012 (Kim et al., 2012). Local health jurisdictions in most states also have the authority to enact disease control measures, including imposing isolation, in response to reports of TB (CDC, 2012).

Immigrant, Refugee, and Migrant Screening Responsibilities

In addition to supporting efforts to curb the spread of infectious disease at U.S. ports of entry, the DGMQ is also responsible for preventing the importation of infectious diseases into the United States by protecting the health of incoming U.S.-bound immigrants, refugees, and asylum seekers (CDC, 2021e).[17] The DGMQ's Immigrant, Refugee, and Migrant Health (IRMH) Branch[18] works with a range of federal interagency partners, governments, and other organizations to promote the health of immigrants, U.S.-bound refugees, and migrants and to bolster health systems to prevent disease spread across international borders.

HHS has the regulatory authority to promulgate regulations that establish requirements for the medical examination of immigrants, refugees, and nonimmigrants required to have an examination prior to admission to the United States.[19] Under this authority, the DGMQ administers regulations regarding health-related conditions that determine ineligibility for entry into the country. They have established systems for cohorts, such as overseas screening programs, treatment protocols, and vaccination requirements (Ortega et al., 2011). All immigrants and refugees entering the United States receive mandatory medical examinations, which includes TB screening conducted by panel physicians in over 150 countries. In addition, refugees are

---

[17] An immigrant is any individual legally admitted to the United States as a lawful permanent resident. A refugee is defined as "any person who is outside the country of such person's nationality or, in the case of a person having no nationality, is outside any country in which such person last habitually resided. In addition, it is a person who is unable or unwilling to return to, and is unable or unwilling to avail himself or herself of the protection of, that country because of persecution, or a well-founded fear of persecution, on account of race, religion, nationality, membership in a particular social group, or political opinion." A migrant is an individual who temporarily or permanently moves away from their place of usual residence, either within a country or across an international border. An asylum seeker is an individual who is seeking protection within the United States due to having suffered or having a well-founded fear of suffering persecution due to their race, religion, nationality, membership in a particular social group, or political opinion. (Source: https://www.uscis.gov/humanitarian/refugees-and-asylum/asylum, accessed April 29, 2022.)

[18] More information about the work of the Immigrant, Refugee, and Migrant Health (IRMH) Branch is available from https://www.cdc.gov/ncezid/dgmq/focus-areas/irmh.html (accessed March 15, 2022).

[19] Title 8: Aliens and Nationality and Title 42: The Public Health and Welfare of the U.S. Code and relevant supporting regulations at Title 42 Public Health in the Code of Federal Regulations (CFR). (Source: https://www.cdc.gov/immigrantrefugeehealth/laws-regulations.html, accessed March 15, 2022.)

provided with public health interventions such as vaccination and parasitic treatment programs. Health records from these activities are provided to U.S. state and local health departments and screening clinics along with notifications of the arrival of all refugees and the subset of immigrants with health conditions for which medical follow-up is recommended.[20]

As of 2012, four quarantine stations at U.S. ports of entry were responsible for meeting and providing a TB-clinic referral to immigrants who had been diagnosed with admissible TB conditions during their pre-immigration medical examination. A study found that immigrants with noninfectious TB who received such referrals—the costs of which are typically covered by state and local health departments—were about four times more likely to engage in follow-up evaluation than those who did not (Kim et al., 2012). For newly arrived immigrants with prior TB infection or previously treated active disease, follow-up care is particularly critical, due to their heightened risk of developing or redeveloping active disease during the first years after they arrive. In 2018, the DGMQ, in collaboration with U.S. Department of State (DOS), launched the U.S. version of eMedical. This is a system for processing overseas medical examination data for immigrants. Panel physicians in the countries in which the examinations are performed enter data directly into the eMedical system, and the data are transferred to the DGMQ's Electronic Disease Notification system within 2 days of the immigrant's arrival in the United States. The substantial reduction in record-processing time increases the likelihood that health departments will be able to initiate timely follow-up with new-arrival immigrants relative to the earlier paper-based systems (Phares et al., 2022). As a result, the QBHSB staff are less involved with meeting immigrants and refugees since the notifications to health departments are automated.

In 2009, the CDC revised the vaccination criteria for U.S. immigration to align with the criteria for vaccines recommended by the Advisory Committee on Immunization Practices (ACIP) to determine which vaccines are required for immigrants to the United States. According to these vaccination criteria, the vaccine must (1) be age appropriate for the immigrant applicant, (2) protect against a disease that has the potential to cause an outbreak, and (3) protect against a disease that has been or is in the process of being eliminated in the United States.[21] The responsibilities of the IRMH Branch are illustrated in Box 3-1.

---

[20] More information about these activities is available from https://www.cdc.gov/immigrant refugeehealth/about-irmh.html, https://www.cdc.gov/immigrantrefugeehealth/riise-project.html, and https://www.cdc.gov/immigrantrefugeehealth/Electronic-Disease-Notification-System.html (accessed March 15, 2022).

[21] More information about CDC's revised criteria for vaccination for immigration is available from https://www.cdc.gov/immigrantrefugeehealth/laws-regs/vaccination-immigration/revised-vaccination-criteria-immigration.html (accessed March 15, 2022).

BOX 3-1
Responsibilities of the Immigrant, Refugee, and Migrant Health Branch

The Immigrant, Refugee, and Migrant Health (IRMH) Branch prevents the importation of infectious diseases by safeguarding the health of U.S.-bound immigrant and refugee populations. IRMH achieves this by:

- Tracking and responding to disease outbreaks in (1) refugee populations overseas and in the United States and (2) in host countries when the outbreak may cross an international border
- Developing technical instructions and training health care providers who perform mandatory overseas predeparture medical exams to ensure that health conditions are documented and treated as required
- Overseeing the required medical examination of refugee and immigrant visa applicants before they travel to the United States
- Promoting, monitoring, and improving the health of children adopted outside of the United States
- Educating immigrant and refugee groups and partners about disease prevention and good health practices
- Coordinating with domestic health departments, foreign health agencies, and nongovernmental organizations to develop, implement, and evaluate programs that improve health outcomes in globally mobile populations
- Partnering with other governments to provide technical assistance at points of entry, along informal cross-border movement, and for cross-border collaboration building to strengthen surveillance, preparedness, and response among mobile populations
- Promoting preventive treatments for and vaccination of refugees and immigrants before departure for several communicable diseases
- Providing technical assistance and training to regional medical and public health officials allowing them to identify, treat, and track diseases that threaten the health of refugees, immigrants, and U.S. residents

SOURCE: CDC, 2021e.

Land-Border Crossing Responsibilities: U.S.–Mexico Border

The DGMQ's United States–Mexico Unit (U.S. MU) plays a major role in preventing the transmission of infectious diseases across the nation's land-border crossings at the U.S.–Mexico border. To execute these responsibilities, the CDC and DGMQ collaborate with U.S. and Mexico health officials at the local, state, and federal levels to support efforts to (1) limit the cross-border spread of infectious diseases, (2) protect the health of people living in the U.S.–Mexico border region, and (3) promote the health of travelers, migrants, and other mobile populations.[22] Housed within U.S. M.U. is the CureTB program that works with states and local jurisdictions across the United States to assist in continuity of care for mobile patients with tuberculosis who intend to travel outside the United States prior to treatment completion, by linking them to TB services in destination countries. The program also accepts referrals from international sources requesting continuity of care linkages for TB patients planning travel to the United States.[23] CureTB also uses their international connections to assist quarantine stations and the Travel Restriction and Interventions Activity to determine when people can be removed from the DNB list and Public Health Lookout prior to U.S. reentry.

The QBHSB is responsible for preventing the transmission of communicable diseases across the nation's northern border crossings along the U.S.–Canadian border. Although the QBHSB does not have staff physically present along the northern border, these activities are executed remotely by the airport-based quarantine stations located in Boston, MA (BOS), New York, NY (JFK), Detroit, MI (DTW), Minneapolis, MN (MSP), and Seattle, WA (SEA). These specific quarantine stations partner with the CBP and STLT health jurisdictions to ensure plans are in place and understood to provide for consequence management should ill travelers or CDC-regulated goods be detected at the U.S.–Canadian border.

In the United States, people of international origin have a higher rate of TB than the U.S.-born population, with those born in Mexico representing the majority of new TB cases between 1993 and 2015 (DeSisto et al., 2015). In 2015, about two-thirds of TB cases among internationally born individuals occurred in the border states of California, Texas, Arizona, and New Mexico (DeSisto et al., 2015). Given that more than 159 million individuals entered the United States at the land-border crossing with Mexico in 2012, for example, the U.S.–Mexico interface creates prime conditions for the transmission of TB across the border, which requires coordinated cross-border follow-up and control strategies (DeSisto et al., 2015).

A study evaluated the use of DNB and Lookout lists to detect and refer back to treatment individuals with infectious or potentially infectious TB crossing the U.S.–Mexico land border between 2007 and 2013 (DeSisto et al., 2015). Most cases were Hispanic, male citizens of the United States or Mexico, more than 30 percent of whom were undocumented migrants and about 20 percent of whom had MDR-TB. Nearly two-thirds of the cases were located and treated due to their placement on the list, but about

---

[22] More information about the work of DGMQ's U.S.–Mexico Unit is available at https://www.cdc.gov/ncezid/dgmq/focus-areas/usmh.html (accessed March 16, 2022).

[23] More information on the CureTB Program is available from https://www.cdc.gov/usmexicohealth/curetb.html (accessed May 10, 2022).

one-quarter—mainly undocumented migrants—were lost to follow-up. The authors suggested several strategies to improve the effectiveness of the Public Health Lookout tool at the U.S.–Mexico border, including (1) using the tool earlier for binational individuals who are at risk of progressing to infectious TB due to treatment nonadherence and are likely to travel across the border, (2) training U.S. CBP officers to contact the CDC if they locate undocumented migrants who are on the Public Health Lookout, and (3) collaborating with Immigration and Customs Enforcement (ICE) on TB referral projects and resources (DeSisto et al., 2015).

Maritime Responsibilities

The maritime industry presents unique public health challenges due to the thousands of ships that make calls at U.S. ports each year, the number of passengers on cruise ships, and crew members often arriving from countries with suboptimal vaccination coverage (CDC, 2011). The CDC is responsible for addressing disease outbreaks on both cruise ships and noncruise ships. Federal regulations authorize the CDC to conduct public health prevention measures at U.S. ports of entry to prevent the introduction and spread of communicable diseases. The agency issues guidance and orders for ships to follow in reducing the risk of disease transmission and in responding to illnesses suggestive of communicable diseases (CDC, 2020, 2022c). International conveyances traveling to the United States are required to report all onboard deaths and illnesses meeting the CDC's regulatory definition to the CDC (CDC, 2021b). Between 2010 and 2014, the DGMQ's quarantine stations received almost 3,000 individual maritime case reports of illnesses (77 percent of reports) and deaths (23 percent) (Stamatakis et al., 2017). The most frequent illness reported was varicella (36 percent) and the most common causes of death were cardiovascular or pulmonary-related conditions (80 percent).

In September and October of 2019 the CDC's Vessel Sanitation Program was notified of three outbreaks of acute gastroenteritis that proved to be norovirus on cruise ships (Rispens et al., 2020). The CDC surveyed passengers, collected and tested specimens to confirm norovirus, partnered with the Food and Drug Administration (FDA) to test food samples for the virus, and determined the source of contamination from a berry supplier in China. Cruises continued to operate as normal during the outbreak, and no known land transmission was reported to be linked. The CDC coordinates CaliciNet, a national network of federal, state, and local public health laboratories that conduct norovirus surveillance activities (CDC, 2019b).

As discussed in Chapter 5, the CDC coordinated a number of mitigation efforts during the COVID-19 pandemic. On March 14, 2020, a No Sail Order issued by the CDC went into effect (CDC, 2022g) that ceased operations of cruise ships in waters under U.S. jurisdiction. The order also required cruise ship operators to develop comprehensive plans for preventing, monitoring, and responding to COVID-19. On October 30, 2020, the CDC lifted the No Sail Order and instituted the Framework for Conditional Sailing Order that was in place from November 1, 2020, to January 15, 2022. This framework involved a phased approach of testing, screening, and simulation measures required to obtain a COVID-19 Conditional Sailing Certificate. The certificate would enable a cruise ship operator to resume passenger operations. On January 29, 2021, the CDC issued an order requiring that all people—including both passengers and employees—on public transportation conveyances or on the premises of transportation hubs wear face masks (*Federal Register*, 2021). In February 2022 all cruise lines were required to either participate or formally opt out of the CDC COVID-19 Program for Cruise Ships (CDC, 2022b). This program provides travelers with color-coded status for cruise ships to inform travel choices. Travelers can review data such as the number of COVID-19 cases a ship has reported, the public health measures a ship is taking, and whether a ship warranted investigation or has opted out of the program.

Responsibilities for Animals

The DGMQ is responsible for regulating the entry of certain animals and products of animal origin into the United States and restricting animal products that could be harmful to humans (CDC, 2021f). Quarantine stations are charged with inspecting CDC-regulated animals and animal products that pose a potential threat to human health. For example, in 2021 the CDC suspended the importation of dogs from 113 countries classified as being at high risk for dog rabies after experiencing an increase in the number of canines arriving with incomplete vaccination documentation (CDC, 2022e; Cima, 2021). The CDC has estimated that approximately 1.06 million dogs are imported into the United States each year, with 700,000 arriving via air travel and 360,000 at land-border ports of entry. The CDC and U.S. Department of Agriculture (USDA) both regulate the entry of dogs, with the USDA and CBP being the only agencies that track the purpose of importation for a subset of dogs. The CDC requires all dogs arriving in the United States to be healthy upon arrival. Additionally, dogs from countries at high risk for canine rabies virus variant are denied entry if they arrive without proper documentation of rabies vaccination or without a CDC-issued permit. The USDA has additional regulations if the intent of importation is for resale purposes (USDA, 2019). Additionally, the DGMQ carries out federal quarantine regulations that prohibit the importation of nonhuman primates as pets due to their ability to transmit TB and other pathogens to humans (CDC, 2022a). All nonhuman primates that enter the United States are inspected by the DGMQ, with 33,818 nonhuman primates imported in FY2019 (Galland, 2021). All nonhuman primates imported into the United States are held in a CDC-approved quarantine facility for at least 31 days and are tested for TB and monitored for symptoms of disease. If a nonhuman primate dies during the quarantine period, the cause of death will be determined through an animal autopsy and series of diagnostic tests (CDC, 2022d). The CDC prohibited the importation of rodents of African origin into the United States due to an importation-related outbreak of monkeypox in 2003 (CDC, 2015a). The CDC also regulates the importation of bats,[24] turtles,[25] and civets[26] due to the association these animals have with previous outbreaks of disease in human populations.

To this date, there is no evidence suggesting that animals play a significant role in the transmission of the SARS-CoV-2 virus to humans. However, studies show that many animals can be infected with the virus although reported transmission from animals to humans have been rare.[27] Future studies are needed to further investigate the transmission of the virus from animals to humans. Modeling studies could be utilized to better understand possible scenarios of transmission. There is the potential that canine and other exotic pet imports will increase due to the growing U.S. demand. Therefore, continued vigilance will be essential with the possibility of new zoonotic disease threats emerging beyond canine rabies.

Human Remains

The CDC regulates the importation of biologics and human remains, which are coregulated by the Division of Select Agents and Toxins (DSAT) and the DGMQ. The DGMQ will respond to inquiries at ports of entry for biologic shipments (any shipment containing human or CDC-regulated animal tissues, body fluids, blood, etc.) and human remains that do not meet U.S. importation requirements, such as those with inadequate documentation or packaging violations. In 2020, the DGMQ and the DSAT updated the human remains importation regulation to provide clarification regarding the definition of human remains and that hermetically sealed caskets were no longer required as long as the remains were packaged in a leak-proof container.[28]

---

[24] https://www.cdc.gov/importation/bringing-an-animal-into-the-united-states/bats.html (accessed May 10, 2022).
[25] https://www.cdc.gov/importation/bringing-an-animal-into-the-united-states/turtles.html (accessed May 10, 2022).
[26] https://www.cdc.gov/importation/bringing-an-animal-into-the-united-states/civets.html (accessed May 10, 2022).
[27] https://www.cdc.gov/coronavirus/2019-ncov/daily-life-coping/animals.html (accessed May 10, 2022).
[28] More information about CDC's human remains importation requirements is available at https://www.cdc.gov/importation/human-remains.html (accessed May 10, 2022).

The DGMQ's Emergency Response Activities

The DGMQ's network of quarantine stations and existing partnerships with federal, STLT, and international agencies and public health authorities is envisioned to scale to support emergency responses to emerging and ongoing infectious disease threats within the United States and abroad.[29]

In situations of a localized outbreak of concern in another country or region of the world, the DGMQ supports the CDC's efforts to stop outbreaks where they begin and help prevent infectious diseases from spreading across borders. In response to the West Africa Ebola outbreak (2014–2016), the DGMQ deployed personnel to support border health measures to reduce the risk of exportation and translocation of disease.[30] Specifically, the DGMQ provided technical support to strengthen airport exit screening for outbound travelers in the Ebola-affected countries. These activities were conducted in coordination with those countries, the World Health Organization, and the International Organization for Migration. After two case importations into the United States, the DGMQ worked with the DHS to conduct public health risk assessments of incoming travelers from the Ebola-affected countries for travelers funneled to selected airports with CDC Quarantine Stations. At these stations (Atlanta, New York, Newark, Washington, DC-Dulles, and Chicago), CDC and DHS staff conducted reviews of traveler health declaration forms, symptom screening, temperature checks, and visual inspections, and collected contact information that was shared with health departments in destination locations to facilitate recommended post-arrival monitoring.

This is particularly critical for outbreaks that could have hugely deleterious consequences if cases were imported into the United States, such as during the Ebola epidemic in Western Africa in 2014–2015. Diseases with potential or definite pandemic potential, such as a novel influenza strain with early evidence of human–human transmission and COVID-19, represent an even more substantial threat to the health of all populations worldwide, thus supporting a rapid and effective emergency response soon after outbreak detection (CDC, 2021d).

Emergency Response and Active Monitoring for Ebola Epidemic in West Africa

As part of the CDC's response to the Ebola epidemic in West Africa—a major global health emergency—the DGMQ and its quarantine station

---

[29] More information about CDC's emergency response activities is available from https://www.cdc.gov/ncezid/dgmq/emergency-response.html (accessed March 16, 2022).

[30] Travel and Border Health Measures to Prevent the International Spread of Ebola. *MMWR Supplements*, July 8, 2016, 65(3):57–67.

network supported a range of disease control efforts.[31] These included (1) providing screening, monitoring, and outreach to travelers arriving from West Africa, (2) streamlining response efforts by working with federal authorities to divert passengers arriving from high-risk countries to just five U.S. airports, (3) training CBP staff at these five airports to screen travelers arriving from high-risk countries for signs and symptoms of Ebola or possible exposures, and (4) in very close collaboration with state and local public health agencies, developing a program to monitor all arriving travelers for 21 days after their departure (CDC, 2015b).

From 2014 to 2016, 36,059 travelers arriving into the United States from three West African countries—Sierra Leone, Guinea, and Liberia—underwent active monitoring for 21 days after a monitoring system was put in place by the CDC in partnership with state and local health departments (CDC, 2015b).[32] This system was largely a response to the first case of Ebola in an arriving international passenger in Dallas, Texas (CDC, 2014). The diagnosis of Ebola in this individual was delayed for 2 days after initial presentation to the hospital, resulting in transmission to two health care workers (CDC, 2019a). There were no additional Ebola cases detected through this large-scale active monitoring effort during the 15-month period in which this system was in place.

Of the 11 Ebola cases treated in the United States, most were identified in countries in West Africa and flown back to the United States for care (CDC, 2019a). Of the two cases detected after reentry into the United States—which occurred before the active monitoring system was established—the first case in Dallas was not recognized as a potential case until late in the person's illness, as their direct exposure risk to a person with Ebola in West Africa was not identified until that point. The second case, which occurred in New York City, self-identified prior to seeking medical care and at the onset of their symptoms, because the individual had potential exposure through working as a health care provider in an Ebola Treatment Unit in Guinea.[33]

Although no additional cases were detected through this active monitoring program, it had several unintended consequences. Individuals under active monitoring who developed symptoms, such as fever, needed to be evaluated first to rule out Ebola—usually at a designated Ebola assessment or treatment hospital. This practice often delayed testing and care for other serious diseases, especially malaria, which is common among persons returning from Western Africa. An analysis of monitoring and movement

---

[31] More information about DGMQ's emergency response to the Ebola epidemic is available at https://www.cdc.gov/ncezid/dgmq/emergency-response.html (accessed March 16, 2022).

[32] This text was modified after release of the report to the study sponsor to correctly identify the agency with authority over the monitoring system.

[33] This text was modified after release of the report to the study sponsor to clarify the nature of the exposure experienced in the second case.

restriction policies implemented in the United States during the Ebola epidemic (2014–2016) found that movement restriction policies—including quarantine—required substantial resources to implement and varied from voluntary to mandatory programs. Additionally, there was a lack of clarity in some of the quarantine enforcement procedures (Sell et al., 2021) For example, a nurse who returned to the United States in 2014 after working in Sierra Leone was ordered to spend 4 days in isolation followed by 3 weeks of quarantine, despite a lack of any symptoms of illness. A lawsuit followed, resulting in a modification of the 3-week home confinement order. Medical groups opposed these regulations, stating that automatic 3-week quarantines for all travelers returning from Ebola-affected areas, with no regard for symptoms, would discourage health care workers from responding to the Ebola outbreak. Some state health departments, on the other hand, maintained that these regulations were necessary for public health (Price, 2016). This incident highlights the complexities of state interactions in issuing public health orders.

Emergency Response to the COVID-19 Pandemic

At the outset of the COVID-19 pandemic in January 2020, the DGMQ was called on to assist in the CDC's emergency response. Through the response, the DGMQ has supported a wide range of activities, including "providing guidance, recommendations, and requirements; educating travelers and migrant populations; working with international, federal, STLT, and industry partners; and protecting the health of immigrants, migrants, refugees, and communities along U.S. borders" (CDC, 2021d). More information about the DGMQ's emergency response activities during the COVID-19 pandemic is provided in Box 3-2. Simultaneously, the DGMQ also supported response activities for Ebola, resettlement of U.S. citizens and lawful permanent residents as well as vulnerable Afghans, and public health interventions for migrants at the Southwest border.

IMPROVING STRATEGIC PLANNING FOR POTENTIAL DISEASE OUTBREAKS

Experiences during recent emergency response efforts highlight the importance of scenario-based planning for the most likely and/or concerning potential disease outbreaks, with the active involvement of key partners. The committee identified multiple opportunities to improve strategic planning for potential disease outbreaks in the domains of (1) coordinated and collaborative advanced planning, (2) large-scale isolation and quarantine planning, and (3) ethics and equity considerations. The committee also developed a potential prioritization scheme for categorization of pathogens to help inform scenario planning illustrated in Table 3-1.

BOX 3-2
The DGMQ Emergency Response Activities during the COVID-19 Pandemic

- Established public health guidance on the management of domestic and international travelers with potential COVID-19 exposure.
- Published guidance for domestic and international travelers on how to protect themselves and others before, during, and after travel.
- Posted Travel Health Notices to alert travelers and other audiences to COVID-19 health threats around the world and advise them on how to protect themselves—more than 1,000 such notices were posted between January 2020 and June 2021.
- Issued orders and regulatory actions including (1) No Sail and Conditional Sailing Orders to respond to and mitigate the spread of COVID-19 on cruise ships; (2) testing, vaccination, and contact information orders for airplane passengers coming to the United States and mask order for conveyances and transportation hubs; and (3) mass issuance of quarantine orders (and isolation orders for those who tested positive) for repatriated citizens from Wuhan, China (the location of the first outbreak) and passengers from the *Diamond Princess* and *Grand Princess* cruise ships, which had COVID-19 outbreaks early in the pandemic—the first quarantine orders that the CDC had issued since 1963. Each of these actions was unprecedented in CDC history.
- Stood up, staffed, and conducted public health risk assessment for 766,044 air passengers coming to the United States from January through September 2020. Deployed 100 responders in 48 hours, plus 500 additional responders sent to U.S. Quarantine Stations to support the program.
- Worked with CBP on traveler contact data collection and shared info with STLT partners for follow-up.
- Supported travel restrictions (Do Not Board and Public Health Lookout lists).
- Supported contact investigations throughout the pandemic including for infections caused by variants of concern.
- Launched the COVID-19 Travel Planner, a crowdsourced web platform in which health departments could upload jurisdiction-specific recommendations and requirements to help travelers learn about travel recommendations and requirements at their U.S. destinations; make informed decisions; protect themselves; and reduce virus transmission before, during, and after domestic travel.
- Developed and disseminated extensive messaging, including Travel Health Alert Notices given to international travelers arriving at major U.S. airports (over 6 million distributed), messages on digital airport monitors, public service announcements for travelers, tool kits for road travel and airline partners, and resources in more than 30 languages to reach people in their native languages.
- Worked to protect newly resettled and long-term resident refugees, immigrants, and migrants, including agricultural workers, and to provide them with culturally and linguistically appropriate resources.
- Monitored and responded to outbreaks of COVID-19 in refugee camps in Africa and Asia.
- Established a pilot genomic surveillance program for SARS-CoV-2 variants at the U.S. ports of entry and rapidly expanded it after identification of the Omicron variant.

SOURCE: CDC, 2021d.

TABLE 3-1 Potential Prioritization Scheme for Categorization of Pathogens

Category	Description of Categorized Pathogens
Primary	The focus of this category would be on pathogens of highest public health importance that are absent from the United States or that do not yet have sustained transmission in the United States but that can cause large or impactful outbreaks with public health and/or economic consequences in the United States if introduced. Examples include novel and reemerging respiratory pathogens, especially viruses, of pandemic or significant public health consequence not yet in the United States; novel and reemerging other pathogens, especially viruses, of significant public health consequence not presently in or with sustained transmission in the United States (e.g., viral hemorrhagic fevers).
Secondary	The focus of this category would be on pathogens present in the United States but whose transmission is facilitated by the act of travel or exposures during travel; examples include measles in congregant settings during maritime travel, infectious TB during air travel, highly drug-resistant pathogens including those in individuals who sought medical care overseas, and highly transmissible pathogens associated with group settings during travel, especially those that can spread readily among at-risk or unvaccinated populations (examples would include measles, meningitis, varicella).
Tertiary	The focus of this category should be on pathogens with individual or limited risk of spread in the United States (e.g., XDR-TB), and pathogens already present and with sustained transmission in the United States.

Coordinated and Collaborative Advanced Planning

As will be discussed in Chapter 5, an evaluation of reporting ill travelers to the QBHSB established a set of recommendations for the CDC and QBHSB, many of which highlight the importance of collaborative planning in advance (Council of State and Territorial Epidemiologists, 2019):

- "Develop standardized protocols/algorithms for jurisdiction reporting to quarantine stations.
- Provide clarity and justification for each piece of data requested for reporting a case.
- Distribute the QBHSB annual report to jurisdictions.
- Hold annual meetings and drills between quarantine stations and jurisdictions in the region covered by each station.
- Develop a training webinar and downloadable reference document with information essential for jurisdiction reporting to DGMQ/QBHSB.
- Explore additional opportunities for communication with state, local, and territorial health departments."

Planning for Large-Scale Isolation and Quarantine

Experiences during past outbreaks, epidemics, and pandemics of infectious diseases have underscored the critical need for large-scale isolation and quarantine planning, as well the consequences of the failure to plan. It is also critical to engage in collaborative advance planning to develop approaches to support continuity of care for individuals after arrival in the United States—particularly for at-risk or vulnerable populations.

For instance, the responses to the Ebola virus disease outbreaks in Western Africa (2014–2016), as well as the COVID-19 pandemic, were undermined by lack of planning to identify potential sites and operational needs to support the large-scale isolation and quarantine measures required for effective management of international passengers with illness and/or exposures. There were gaps in clarity of standards or predetermined roles and responsibilities around housing infrastructure and wraparound services, including issues related to transportation between facilities or jurisdictions. Across different jurisdictions, there was substantial variation in their respective capacities to offer resources (Allen, 2022). Moreover, there was a lack of clarity extending throughout the federal, state, local, tribal, and territorial levels regarding which entities had various authorities and when, as well as ambiguity about their respective roles and responsibilities. Additionally, there was wide variation in state and local implementation of quarantine and isolation measures (Allen, 2022).

The Association of State and Territorial Health Officials (ASTHO) has suggested strategies to strengthen isolation and quarantine preparedness planning: (1) define federal, state, and local roles and responsibilities; (2) evaluate plans through drills and exercises with stakeholders; and (3) develop tools to estimate resource costs for isolation and quarantine. They have also suggested evaluating the use of direct active monitoring to determine when it is appropriate (e.g., its effectiveness may be limited for respiratory illnesses), to understand resource requirements, and to explore opportunities to leverage virtual technologies if appropriate.

Ethics and Equity Considerations

As will be discussed in Chapter 4, the committee identified a set of key ethical principles for consideration in disease control measures and innovations. These foundational principles also apply to the implementation of large-scale quarantine and isolation and include (1) protecting privacy, (2) maintaining autonomy, (3) promoting equity, (4) minimizing the risk of error, and (5) ensuring accountability.

Disease control efforts by their nature need to include ethics, privacy, and equity considerations. The infringement on individual rights to maximize public health benefits should only take place when deemed necessary, effective, and proportional to the threat, and within a context of supportive services to provide shelter, food, medicine, and other basic needs, and should be as limited and of as short a duration as necessary to maximally effect the desired outcome (Rothstein, 2015). The effects of quarantine on individuals can be substantial. Time spent in isolation can result in significant loss of income, which can be detrimental—and in some cases devastating—for individuals (Nuffield Council on Bioethics, 2020; WHO, 2016). A literature review found that the psychological impact of quarantine can be substantial, wide ranging, and long lasting (Brooks et al., 2020). Experiences and stressors related to quarantine included posttraumatic stress symptoms, confusion, anger, fear, financial loss, and stigma. Given that isolation and quarantine can cause or exacerbate mental health concerns, mental health supports need to be considered when these disease control measures are deemed necessary (Nakazawa et al., 2020). For example, when passengers were quarantined for 14 days after detection of COVID-19 cases aboard a cruise ship in March 2020, they were provided with smartphones that could be used to access free health consultations and place medication requests. Enabling quarantined individuals to communicate with loved ones via provision of internet access and devices can also reduce feelings of isolation, stress, and panic (Brooks et al., 2020). It is also important to address the special needs of certain quarantined populations (including children, older adults, and people with disabilities) to ensure that the services they receive are culturally and linguistically appropriate. This includes ensuring that personnel are available to assist individuals who may have difficulty navigating these technologies.

BORDER MEASURES AND ACTIVE MONITORING OF INTERNATIONAL TRAVELERS DURING COVID-19: EVALUATION

The committee evaluated research on the effectiveness of border measures and active monitoring of international travelers during COVID-19. Overall, the effectiveness of border measures, including pretravel testing, is unclear, and additional research is needed to determine the factors that contribute to successful screening measures. Overall, evidence suggests that border and screening measures may be more effective when used within the context of a national disease mitigation program and not relied on as the sole mechanism for reducing transmission.

Effectiveness of Border Screening

Border screening is the process by which incoming travelers are tested or otherwise assessed for signs of illness. In the United States, the DGMQ partners with U.S. CBP to provide enhanced screening for incoming travelers, including symptom screening for COVID-19, both at airports and the southern border (Rasicot, 2021).[34] In many countries, much of the research on border screening involved polymerase chain reaction (PCR) or antigen testing before traveling and/or after arrival. Both modeling and empirical studies provide evidence of the potential effectiveness of border screening in reducing the transmission of COVID-19. Results from one modeling study suggest that, when used as a solitary measure, a single-test screening process before departure was not sufficient to prevent a local outbreak at the arrival destination, because it had not been found to significantly reduce the number of infected travelers entering a country (Bays et al., 2021). A study conducted in Iceland found that COVID-19 testing conducted twice post-arrival reduced the risk of false-negative results that can lead to the spread of infection (Baddal et al., 2021). While more research is needed, initial studies suggest that a single test may not be a strong-enough border screening measure to reduce the spread of COVID-19.

One study conducted an international meta-analysis of both modeling and observational studies and stated that both types have reported mixed results when assessing the effectiveness of COVID-19 screening measures (Burns et al., 2021). Modeling studies found that COVID-19 screening based on symptoms or potential exposure reduced imported or exported cases and delayed outbreaks; however, the authors expressed concerns with the quality of some models, noting inconsistencies in assumptions and parameters. (Burns et al., 2021). Modeling studies predicted that this form of screening would detect between 1 and 53 percent of infected travelers. Observational studies reported a wide range of positive cases detected—between 0 to 100 percent—with the majority of studies reporting fewer than 54 percent of cases detected. For screening based on testing rather than on symptoms or potential exposure, modeling studies reported that testing travelers reduced both imported or exported cases and cases detected. Observational studies reported that the proportion of cases detected varied from 58 to 90 percent, with variability potentially being attributable to timing of testing (Burns et al., 2021). An observational study concluded that COVID-19 border screening by testing can involve very low positive predictive values and high costs per positive case detected (Grunér et al., 2022). A Bayesian modeling approach to estimate the relative capacity for detection of imported cases of COVID-19 for 194 locations (excluding China) compared with that for Singapore estimated the ability to detect Wuhan-to-location imported cases of COVID-19 to be 38 percent (Niehus et al., 2020).

---

[34] This text was modified after release of the report to the study sponsor to clarify the division's role and responsibilities.

As part of California's efforts to reduce introductions of COVID-19 into the state and country during the initial months of the COVID-19 pandemic, the state implemented a program to screen travelers from selected countries on entry and to obtain their contact information and share it with other states for monitoring purposes. Despite this very labor-intensive effort, this traveler screening system did not effectively prevent the introduction of COVID-19 into California. In California, barriers to effective COVID-19 monitoring and screening of travelers included incomplete traveler information transmitted to federal officials and states, the number of travelers requiring follow-up, and potential presymptomatic and asymptomatic transmission (Myers et al., 2020).[35] This suggests that during an outbreak, health departments have to be cautious about devoting their often-limited resources to these types of monitoring efforts, rather than channeling those resources into more effective mitigation strategies.

During the early phases of the COVID-19 pandemic, the CDC also implemented an entry screening program at certain airports for passengers arriving from designated countries (Dollard et al., 2020). This effort required substantial resources, yet the yield of laboratory-confirmed COVID-19 cases was low (1 case per 85,000 travelers screened) and—because it was conducted with manual data collection—contact information was missing for a substantial proportion of travelers who were screened. The low case-detection rate of this resource-intensive program highlighted the need for fundamental change in the U.S. border health strategy. For a disease such as COVID-19, with nonspecific clinical presentation and asymptomatic cases, symptom-based screening programs are not effective. More effective strategies for mitigating the importation of COVID-19 cases could include (1) enhanced communication with travelers regarding preventive measures, and (2) expanding predeparture and post-arrival testing (Dollard et al., 2020). COVID-19 also presents a unique situation in that early diagnostics were used under emergency use authorizations, and later assessment by the FDA revealed that different tests had different levels of sensitivity in detecting the SARS-CoV-2 virus (FDA, 2020). The effectiveness of a screening measure is dependent on multiple factors, including the characteristics of disease presentation and availability of accurate diagnostics.

---

[35] Biodetection dogs may increase the ability to detect asymptomatic cases. A study found that utilizing biodetection dogs as a preliminary SARS-CoV-2 screening method resulted in an average sensitivity of 82.63 percent (Baddal et al., 2021). The authors noted that PCR testing would be used to confirm identification of infection.

Effectiveness of Strategies to Reduce Case Importation

Evidence suggests that mandatory testing, both before departure and upon arrival, increases accuracy in case detection compared to predeparture testing alone. Repeated testing for travelers quarantined on arrival can also enable shorter quarantine times without increasing the risk of disease spread (Dickens et al., 2021). Travel restrictions are useful in preventing infection spread in the early stages of an outbreak when it is confined to a particular area (Gwee et al., 2021; Kraemer et al., 2020). These restrictions may be less effective once an outbreak spreads to additional locations. Local mitigation strategies are effective in containing both local transmission and more widespread outbreaks.

Modeling studies indicated that testing travelers at entry and isolating those who test positive can achieve similar reductions in disease transmission compared to quarantining all travelers (Dickens et al., 2020). A modeling study found that relative to no screening on entry, testing all incoming travelers and isolating those who tested positive for COVID-19 reduced case importation across countries by 90.2 percent for a 7-day isolation period followed by a negative test and by 91.7 percent for a 14-day isolation followed by a negative test. Isolation for all travelers followed by entry permission without subsequent testing resulted in reductions of case importation of 55.4 percent for 7-day isolation and 91.2 percent for 14-day isolation. Testing all travelers and denying entry to those who tested positive reduced case importation by 77.6 percent.

Vaccine-related measures—such as requiring travelers to be fully or partially vaccinated—reduced the likelihood of importing cases (Ronksley et al., 2021). A study of international travelers arriving by air in Alberta, Canada, in January–February 2021 found that 0.02 percent of travelers who were fully or partially vaccinated against COVID-19 tested positive for the virus, in comparison with 1.42 percent of unvaccinated travelers, although both were relatively low.

Effectiveness of Travel Restrictions

Early detection and isolation of cases have the potential to prevent more infections than targeted travel restrictions and contact reductions, whereas a combination of the aforementioned nonpharmaceutical intervention (NPI) approaches can achieve the strongest and most rapid effect (Lai et al., 2020). Genomic epidemiology analyses of SARS-CoV-2 in China's Guangdong province indicate that large-scale surveillance and NPI were effective in containing the epidemic and limiting dissemination to other provinces (Lu et al., 2020). Europe and the United States were reactive in issuing country-specific travel restrictions only after local transmission of

SARS-CoV-2 was confirmed (Davis et al., 2021). In January and February 2020, testing capacity was limited and restricted to people who had recently traveled to China. Broader testing can bolster local outbreak prevention efforts in providing opportunities for earlier detection and interventions.

Complete border closures only with specific target countries can modestly affect an epidemic's trajectory. More significant containment is achieved when travel restrictions are combined with community mitigation strategies to prevent local transmission (Kwok et al., 2021). Complete border closures in Hong Kong reduced both the cumulative COVID-19 case number and mortality by approximately 14 percent. A modeling study of COVID-19 prevalence in Italy found spatial heterogeneity in the effect of travel restrictions, with regions farthest from the initial outbreak receiving greater benefit from these restrictions (Parino et al., 2021).

The inflow volume of passengers, local case incidence, and local epidemic growth need to be considered when implementing travel restrictions. A modeling study found that many countries can attain a negligible number of imported cases—less than 1 percent—with only selective travel restrictions imposed (Russell et al., 2021). In the early stages of a pandemic, travel restrictions can reduce approximately 80 percent of exportation events (Chinazzi et al., 2020; Wells et al., 2020). This can provide cities unaffected by an outbreak with time to coordinate an appropriate public health response. Research studies indicate benefits of travel restrictions on delaying the spread of outbreaks, but different studies indicated varying lengths of delay ranging from 1 day to 85 days (Burns et al., 2021). Studies found very low–certainty evidence that travel restrictions reduced COVID-19 cases within a community and cases imported or exported. Research indicates that travel restrictions may provide short-term benefits, but these restrictions are ineffective at completely eliminating disease (Aleta et al., 2020). Furthermore, international travel restrictions become ineffective after the early stages of a pandemic (Askitas et al., 2021).

Summary of Evaluation

To prevent or minimize disease transmission in the United States, the committee found questionable evidence for the effectiveness of travel restrictions and border closures for COVID-19 reactively targeting countries only after local transmission is confirmed. More evidence is needed on the potential benefits of these methods. In addition, monitoring of *all* international travelers arriving from outbreak-affected countries, regardless of symptoms or history of exposure, has been shown to be porous to asymptomatic cases. Similar lack of evidence has been documented for pandemic influenza (Bajardi et al., 2011; Cowling et al., 2010; Hollingsworth et al., 2006). Travel restrictions, border closures, and active monitoring of international travelers work best for diseases that have low proportions of asymptomatic and presymptomatic transmission risk and longer incubation periods (Fraser et al., 2004; Hollingsworth et al., 2006). Furthermore, the key to the impact of travel restrictions is the rate of growth of the epidemic in the source country and early implementation of the policies. Travel restrictions and border closure, however, can delay the progression of the epidemic, allowing more time for health authorities to prepare mitigation and control policies. More severe and stringent strategies, such as closing travel to everyone regardless of the country that they are traveling from, may be effective in stopping or slowing the spread of disease, although the economic, social, and political trade-offs of these policies should be carefully evaluated.

For diseases like SARS and Ebola, these interventions are more effective when measures can be more directly targeted to those with known risk exposures, as opposed to targeting all travelers from a country or region. Quarantine with active monitoring of persons at risk and/or exposed works best when most secondary cases become symptomatic after they are separated from others; this helps to prevent ongoing transmission to others (i.e., tertiary cases). These tools were successfully used with SARS and during prior Ebola outbreaks within Africa to stop ongoing transmission—even before a vaccine became available—as well as historically, for diseases like smallpox (Bogoch et al., 2015; Hollingsworth et al., 2006). Both Ebola and smallpox have longer incubation periods and persons are most infectious after they have been symptomatic for several days. It should be noted that travel restrictions and border closures might be needed especially in the early phases of a pandemic when etiology, exact modes of transmission, incubation periods, and other characteristics of novel viruses are unknown.

Detailed analysis concerning the impact of the timing and extent of travel restrictions—that is, number of countries, citizenship, residential status—with respect to the pathogen of interest needs to inform future strategies. Such analysis, through formal evaluation, can help determine the parameters for when these tools should be considered in the future, especially for a highly transmissible respiratory virus with a short incubation period and a high proportion of asymptomatic infections and contagiousness prior to illness onset.

When COVID-19 first emerged in early 2020, its etiology was initially unknown. It took months to start to understand the epidemiologic (i.e., transmission) and clinical characteristics of the SARS-CoV-2 virus to help guide public health measures. However, it then became clear that SARS-CoV-2 had a short incubation period of 2–14 days (with median of 5 days)—especially for more recent variants such as Omicron—as well as a relatively high proportion of asymptomatic persons among confirmed cases (40 percent), with transmission risk occurring among both presymptomatic and asymptomatic cases (Ma et al., 2021). These findings call into question the role of quarantine and active monitoring in minimizing transmission, given the large degree of unrecognized chains of transmission.

Moreover, once COVID-19 transmission was established in the United States, the role of active monitoring of all international travelers from countries deemed at higher risk—many of whom were not symptomatic or likely infected—probably had questionable impact on transmission levels in the United States. However, diverting state and local health department resources to monitor international travelers impacted other local infection control priorities, including vaccination, testing, and outbreak response. Similarly, by the time a new variant of concern of a virus as transmissible as SARS-CoV-2 is recognized overseas, it is likely that it is already widely spreading in other settings. Therefore, the impact of targeted country-level travel restrictions in preventing or minimizing SARS-CoV-2 transmission in the United States was minimal. This was demonstrated in the failed effort against the Omicron variant, when travel bans for selected countries in Africa did not prevent a major pandemic wave from occurring in the United States or elsewhere. The initial travel bans enacted against South Africa and other African countries were decried as discriminatory, as countries in Europe also had reported cases. Travel bans can produce unintended effects, such as placing undue economic burdens on target countries and discouraging researchers from reporting new strains. It is important that travel restrictions are considered within the broader context of the national response, as these restrictions alone are unlikely to be effective in reducing disease spread (WHO, 2021). Lessons learned during recent outbreak and pandemic responses—such as for Ebola and COVID-19—can be keys to guiding policy decisions for when to consider travel restrictions/border closures and active monitoring of international passengers for future pandemics as a tool for minimizing or preventing transmission of diseases in the United States. It should be noted that the current science on the effectiveness on travel restrictions and border closures is not definitive. There is a need for more extensive analyses to better identify and evaluate the methods that were most effective during the COVID-19 pandemic. The DGMQ has a tool kit of options available, and each individual threat should be assessed to determine the best course of action for disease mitigation strategies.

The CDC could also leverage academic partners (see Chapter 5), or the new Center for Forecasting and Outbreak Analytics (see Box 3-3), to provide modeling expertise to help determine the transmission characteristics of microbial pathogens (e.g., median/range of incubation period, proportion of asymptomatic cases and degree of asymptomatic/presymptomatic transmission risk) as well as the outbreak scenarios (e.g., isolated to one country or region) where border restrictions/active monitoring may have the most impact for preventing or minimizing disease introduction into the United States during future pandemics or outbreaks of concern.

> **BOX 3-3**
> **The CDC Center for Forecasting and Outbreak Analytics**
>
> In August 2021, the Centers for Disease Control and Prevention (CDC) announced the establishment of the Center for Forecasting and Outbreak Analytics to advance the use of forecasting and outbreak analytics in public health decision making by bringing together next-generation public health data, expert disease modelers, public health emergency responders, and high-quality communications. The Center will (1) accelerate access to and use of data for public health decision makers who need information to mitigate the effects of disease threats (e.g., social and economic disruption), (2) prioritize equity and accessibility, and (3) serve as a hub for innovation and research on disease modeling.
> The Center will focus on three key functions: predict, connect, and inform.
>
> 1. Predict: Undertake modeling and forecasting; enhance the ability to determine the foundational data sources needed; support research and innovation in outbreak analytics and science for real-time action; and establish appropriate forecasting horizons.
> 2. Connect: Expand broad capability for data sharing and integration; maximize interoperability with data standards and utilize open-source software and application programming interface capabilities, with existing and new data streams from the public health ecosystem and beyond.
> 3. Inform: Translate and communicate forecasts; connect with key decision makers across sectors including government, businesses, and nonprofits, along with individuals with strong intergovernmental affairs and communication capacity for action.
>
> SOURCE: CDC, 2021a.

CONCLUSIONS AND RECOMMENDATIONS

Conclusions

Conclusion 3-1: The DGMQ will benefit from having detailed operational plans/playbooks based on lessons learned from COVID-19 and other recent emergencies (e.g., Ebola viral disease) for the most concerning/likely scenarios for imported disease threats. These operational plans will benefit from feedback from key partners, including state, tribal, local, and territorial public health agencies.

Conclusion 3-2: Planning for larger-scale isolation and quarantine operations has been insufficient—as evidenced in the initial response to COVID-19 in spring 2020—in addressing the need for mass repatriation of U.S. citizens traveling overseas, as well as travelers on cruise ships when COVID-19 outbreaks occur.

Conclusion 3-3: It will be critical to incorporate ethical and equity considerations when implementing border closure measures and placing persons in isolation and quarantine facilities, given their varying effects across different types of travelers (e.g., U.S. travelers returning home, foreign nationals, immigrants/refugees).

Conclusion 3-4: Quarantine and active monitoring of all international travelers coming into the United States—regardless of their symptom status or exposure history—once COVID-19 transmission was occurring nationwide was likely not effective in minimizing transmission in the United States. Furthermore, these measures diverted public health resources from other critical activities.

Conclusion 3-5: Incorporation of research, investigation, modeling, and evaluations in the DGMQ's mission will help to identify optimal interventions and programs to support that mission.

Recommendations

Recommendation 3-1: The Division of Global Migration and Quarantine (DGMQ) should develop detailed operational plans and playbooks based on the most concerning and likely scenarios for transmissible disease threats.
  A. The DGMQ should develop operational plans for the most probable scenarios that are likely to have major impacts requiring disease control interventions based on priority pathogens. These plans should list required partners, enumerate possible response steps, define possible implementation go–no go decision points, and include metrics to assess containment.
  B. The DGMQ should seek input from key agencies and organizations (e.g., the World Health Organization, the Coalition for Epidemic Preparedness Innovations, the U.S. Agency for International Development, the new Centers for Disease Control and Prevention (CDC) Center for Forecasting and Outbreak Analytics, the CDC Center for Public Health Preparedness and Response, and the Office of the Assistant Secretary for Preparedness and Response) as well as state and local public health agencies when determining which pathogens and scenarios to prioritize for planning purposes.

Recommendation 3-2: The Division of Global Migration and Quarantine, in coordination with appropriate federal partners for implementa-

tion, should develop detailed operational plans for large-scale isolation and quarantine needs for future emergencies. These operational plans should be informed by the lessons learned during the initial response to COVID-19. Critical issues to address include:
   A. Potential sites for large-scale isolation and quarantine facilities should be identified in all U.S. Department of Health and Human Services regions. Memoranda of agreement for these facilities should be established prior to any possible need to facilitate rapid setup during a public health emergency. Minimum standards of infrastructure should be established for these facilities including capacity to provide wraparound services, such as health care services, diverse dietary needs, laundry facilities, communication needs, business support services, and entertainment.
   B. Ethical and equity issues that will likely arise, especially when housing/caring for special populations, including families with young children, the elderly, persons with special medical needs, persons with disabilities, refugees, persons who cross borders on a routine basis for work, and persons with pets. The plans should also address language and incorporate intercultural components, normalizing these needs as an expected component of the public health response.
   C. Those plans also need to include
      1. coordination of legal authority and enforcement;
      2. triage, transport, and assessment of ill persons with nearby health care facilities or onsite, available health care personnel; and
      3. collaboration with state and local public health, law enforcement, and emergency management officials.

Recommendation 3-3: The Division of Migration and Quarantine/Centers for Disease Control and Prevention should commission an external formal evaluation and/or a modeling study of the effectiveness of travel restrictions and active screening/monitoring of all international travelers in preventing and mitigating disease transmission in the United States during both the current COVID-19 pandemic and the 2014–2015 Ebola outbreaks in West Africa. The formal evaluation should include psychological benefits, political implications, unintended consequences of screening, resources required, and burden placed on state and local jurisdictions. These findings should be used to inform plans detailing when such measures should be considered in the future and to specify the types of pathogens and scenarios that warrant these measures. The latter criteria might include incubation period, timing of infectiousness related to symptom onset, proportion of asymptomatic infections, size of traveler population that would require monitoring, technological ease and cost of monitoring, severity of illness, and reasonable ability to provide or implement countermeasures.

REFERENCES

Aleta, A., Q. Hu, J. Ye, P. Ji, and Y. Moreno. 2020. A data-driven assessment of early travel restrictions related to the spreading of the novel COVID-19 within mainland China. *Chaos, Solitons and Fractals* 139:110068. https://doi.org/10.1016/j.chaos.2020.110068.

Allen, M. 2022. *Enhancing the Federal Quarantine Station network - A state perspective: ASTHO.* Presentation to the National Academies of Sciences, Engineering, and Medicine Committee on Analysis to Enhance the Effectiveness of the Federal Quarantine Station Network.

Askitas, N., K. Tatsiramos, and B. Verheyden. 2021. Estimating worldwide effects of non-pharmaceutical interventions on COVID-19 incidence and population mobility patterns using a multiple-event study. *Scientific Reports* 11(1):1972. https://dx.doi.org/10.1038/s41598-021-81442-x.

Baddal, B., T. Sanlidag, B. Uzun, and D. Uzun Ozsahin. 2021. The use of double border-screening strategy in the surveillance and prevention of COVID-19. *Journal of Infection and Public Health* 14(6):757-758. https://dx.doi.org/10.1016/j.jiph.2021.03.012.

Bajardi, P., C. Poletto, J. J. Ramasco, M. Tizzoni, V. Colizza, and A. Vespignani. 2011. Human mobility networks, travel restrictions, and the global spread of 2009 H1N1 pandemic. *PLOS ONE* 6(1):e16591. https://doi.org/10.1371/journal.pone.0016591.

Bays, D., E. Bennett, and T. Finnie. 2021. What effect might border screening have on preventing the importation of COVID-19 compared with other infections? A modelling study. *Epidemiology & Infection* 149:e238.

Bogoch, I. I., M. I. Creatore, M. S. Cetron, J. S. Brownstein, N. Pesik, J. Miniota, T. Tam, W. Hu, A. Nicolucci, S. Ahmed, J. W. Yoon, I. Berry, S. I. Hay, A. Anema, A. J. Tatem, D. MacFadden, M. German, and K. Khan. 2015. Assessment of the potential for international dissemination of Ebola virus via commercial air travel during the 2014 West African outbreak. *The Lancet* 385(9962):29-35. https://doi.org/10.1016/s0140-6736(14)61828-6.

Brooks, S. K., R. K. Webster, L. E. Smith, L. Woodland, S. Wessely, N. Greenberg, and G. J. Rubin. 2020. The psychological impact of quarantine and how to reduce it: Rapid review of the evidence. *The Lancet* 395(10227):912-920. https://doi.org/10.1016/s0140-6736(20)30460-8.

Burns, J., A. Movsisyan, J. M. Stratil, R. L. Biallas, M. Coenen, K. M. Emmert-Fees, K. Geffert, S. Hoffmann, O. Horstick, M. Laxy, C. Klinger, S. Kratzer, T. Litwin, S. Norris, L. M. Pfadenhauer, P. von Philipsborn, K. Sell, J. Stadelmaier, B. Verboom, S. Voss, K. Wabnitz, and E. Rehfuess. 2021. International travel-related control measures to contain the COVID-19 pandemic: A rapid review. *Cochrane Database of Systematic Reviews* 3(3):Cd013717. https://doi.org/10.1002/14651858.cd013717.pub2.

CDC (Centers for Disease Control and Prevention). 2011. *Maritime activity.* Atlanta, GA: CDC Division of Global Migration and Quarantine. https://www.cdc.gov/quarantine/pdfs/maritime-industry.pdf (accessed March 15, 2022).

CDC. 2012. *Menu of suggested provisions for state tuberculosis prevention and control laws.* https://www.cdc.gov/tb/programs/laws/menu/enforcement.htm (accessed April 29, 2022).

CDC. 2014. *CDC and Texas Health Department confirm first Ebola case diagnosed in the U.S.* [Press Release]. https://www.cdc.gov/media/releases/2014/s930-ebola-confirmed-case.html (accessed May 18, 2022).
CDC. 2015a. *African rodent importation ban.* https://www.cdc.gov/poxvirus/monkeypox/african-ban.html (accessed March 15, 2022).
CDC. 2015b. *The road to zero: CDC's response to the West African Ebola epidemic 2014–2015. Ebola Report: Protecting Borders.* https://www.cdc.gov/about/ebola/protecting-borders.html#protect (accessed 24 March, 2022).
CDC. 2019a. *2014–2016 Ebola outbreak in West Africa.* https://www.cdc.gov/vhf/ebola/history/2014-2016-outbreak/index.html (accessed March 12, 2022).
CDC. 2019b. *Reporting and surveillance for norovirus: CaliciNet.* https://www.cdc.gov/norovirus/reporting/calicinet/index.html (accessed May 18, 2022).
CDC. 2020. *Cargo ship guidance.* https://www.cdc.gov/quarantine/cargo/index.html (accessed March 12, 2022).
CDC. 2021a. *CDC stands up new disease forecasting center* [Press Release]. https://www.cdc.gov/media/releases/2021/p0818-disease-forecasting-center.html (accessed May 18, 2022).
CDC. 2021b. *Cruise ships: Reporting maritime death or illness (non-gastrointestinal) to DGMQ.* https://www.cdc.gov/quarantine/cruise/reporting-deaths-illness/index.html (accessed March 15, 2022).
CDC. 2021c. *Laws and Regulations.* Division of Global Migration and Quarantine (DGMQ). https://www.cdc.gov/ncezid/dgmq/laws-and-regulations.html (accessed May 18, 2022).
CDC. 2021d. *Emergency response.* Division of Global Migration and Quarantine (DGMQ). https://www.cdc.gov/ncezid/dgmq/emergency-response.html (accessed February 18, 2022).
CDC. 2021e. *Immigrant, Refugee, and Migrant Health Branch.* Division of Global Migration and Quarantine (DGMQ). https://www.cdc.gov/ncezid/dgmq/focus-areas/irmh.html (accessed February 16, 2022).
CDC. 2021f. *Quarantine and border health services.* Division of Global Migration and Quarantine (DGMQ). https://www.cdc.gov/ncezid/dgmq/focus-areas/quarantine.html (accessed February 28, 2022).
CDC. 2022a. *Bringing a nonhuman primate into the United States.* https://www.cdc.gov/importation/bringing-an-animal-into-the-united-states/monkeys.html (accessed March 15, 2022).
CDC. 2022b. *Cruise ship color status.* https://www.cdc.gov/quarantine/cruise/cruise-ship-color-status.html (accessed March 15, 2022).
CDC. 2022c. *Cruise ship guidance.* https://www.cdc.gov/quarantine/cruise/index.html (accessed March 12, 2022).
CDC. 2022d. *FAQs about CDC regulations for the importation of nonhuman primates (NHPs) into the United States.* https://www.cdc.gov/importation/laws-and-regulations/nonhuman-primates/nprm/qa-general.html (accessed March 23, 2022).
CDC. 2022e. *Notice of temporary suspension of dogs entering the United States from countries classified as high risk for dog rabies.* https://www.cdc.gov/importation/bringing-an-animal-into-the-united-states/high-risk-dog-ban-frn.html (accessed March 15, 2022).
CDC. 2022f. *Travel restrictions to prevent the spread of disease.* https://www.cdc.gov/quarantine/travel-restrictions.html (accessed March 12, 2022).
CDC. 2022g. COVID-19 orders for cruise ships. https://www.cdc.gov/quarantine/cruise/covid19-cruiseships.html (accessed March 15, 2022).
CDC and DHS (Department of Homeland Security). 2014. *Fact sheet: Screening of travelers at airports.* https://www.dhs.gov/news/2014/10/08/fact-sheet-screening-travelers-airports (accessed March 24, 2022).

Chinazzi, M., J. T. Davis, M. Ajelli, C. Gioannini, M. Litvinova, S. Merler, Y. P. A. Pastore, K. Mu, L. Rossi, K. Sun, C. Viboud, X. Xiong, H. Yu, M. E. Halloran, I. M. Longini, Jr., and A. Vespignani. 2020. The effect of travel restrictions on the spread of the 2019 novel coronavirus (COVID-19) outbreak. *Science* 368(6489):395-400. https://dx.doi.org/10.1126/science.aba9757.

Cima, G. 2021. CDC eases entry requirements for dogs vaccinated in United States. *JAVMA News*, December 29. https://avmajournals.avma.org/view/post/news/cdc-eases-entry-requirements-for-dogs-vaccinated-in-united-states.xml (accessed May 18, 2022).

Council of State and Territorial Epidemiologists. 2019. *Evaluation of reports of ill travelers to Quarantine and Border Health Services Branch—final report.* https://cdn.ymaws.com/www.cste.org/resource/resmgr/crosscuttingi/Evaluation_of_Reports_of_Ill.pdf (accessed April 15, 2022).

Council of State and Territorial Epidemiologists. 2020. *Notification protocol and data collection guidance: Health department notification to CDC quarantine stations of infectious persons with recent travel.* https://cdn.ymaws.com/www.cste.org/resource/resmgr/crosscuttingi/CSTE_Notification_Protocol_a.pdf (accessed April 15, 2022).

Cowling, B. J., L. L. Lau, P. Wu, H. W. Wong, V. J. Fang, S. Riley, and H. Nishiura. 2010. Entry screening to delay local transmission of 2009 pandemic influenza A (H1N1). *BMC Infectious Diseases* 10(1):1-4. https://doi.org/10.1186/1471-2334-10-82.

Davis, J. T., M. Chinazzi, N. Perra, K. Mu, Y. P. A. Pastore, M. Ajelli, N. E. Dean, C. Gioannini, M. Litvinova, S. Merler, L. Rossi, K. Sun, X. Xiong, I. M. Longini, Jr., M. E. Halloran, C. Viboud, and A. Vespignani. 2021. Cryptic transmission of SARS-CoV-2 and the first COVID-19 wave. *Nature* 600(7887):127-132. https://doi.org/10.1038/s41586-021-04130-w.

DeSisto, C., K. Broussard, M. Escobedo, D. Borntrager, F. Alvarado-Ramy, and S. Waterman. 2015. Border lookout: Enhancing tuberculosis control on the United States-Mexico border. *The American Journal of Tropical Medicine and Hygiene* 93(4):747-751. https://doi.org/10.4269/ajtmh.15-0300.

Dickens, B. L., J. R. Koo, J. T. Lim, H. Sun, H. E. Clapham, A. Wilder-Smith, and A. R. Cook. 2020. Strategies at points of entry to reduce importation risk of COVID-19 cases and reopen travel. *Journal of Travel Medicine* 27(8):taaa141. https://dx.doi.org/10.1093/jtm/taaa141.

Dickens, B. L., J. R. Koo, J. T. Lim, M. Park, H. Sun, Y. Sun, Z. Zeng, S. E. D. Quaye, H. E. Clapham, H. L. Wee, and A. R. Cook. 2021. Determining quarantine length and testing frequency for international border opening during the COVID-19 pandemic. *Journal of Travel Medicine* 28(7):taab088. https://doi.org/10.1093/jtm/taab088.

Dollard, P., I. Griffin, A. Berro, N. J. Cohen, K. Singler, Y. Haber, C. de la Motte Hurst, A. Stolp, S. Atti, L. Hausman, C. E. Shockey, S. Roohi, C. M. Brown, L. D. Rotz, M. S. Cetron, and F. Alvarado-Ramy. 2020. Risk assessment and management of COVID-19 among travelers arriving at designated U.S. Airports, January 17–September 13, 2020. *MMWR: Morbidity and Mortality Weekly Report* 69(45):1681-1685. http://dx.doi.org/10.15585/mmwr.mm6945a4.

FDA (Food and Drug Administration). 2020. *SARS-CoV-2 Reference Panel comparative data.* https://www.fda.gov/medical-devices/coronavirus-COVID-19-and-medical-devices/sars-cov-2-reference-panel-comparative-data (accessed May 6, 2022).

Federal Register. 2021. *Requirement for negative predeparture COVID–19 test result or documentation of recovery from COVID–19 for all airline or other aircraft passengers arriving into the United States from any foreign country* [CDC Notice dated 12/7/2021]. https://www.federalregister.gov/documents/2021/12/07/2021-26603/requirements-for-negative-pre-departure-COVID-19-test-result-or-documentation-of-recovery-from9 (accessed May 18, 2022).

Fraser, C., S. Riley, R. M. Anderson, and N. M. Ferguson. 2004. Factors that make an infectious disease outbreak controllable. *Proceedings of the National Academy of Sciences of the United States of America* 101(16):6146-6151. https://dx.doi.org/10.1073/pnas.0307506101.

Galland, G. 2021. *Presentation on nonhuman primate importation during the SARS-CoV-2 pandemic.* CDC Division of Global Migration and Quarantine. https://www.nationalacademies.org/documents/embed/link/LF2255DA3DD1C41C0A42D3BEF0989A-CAECE3053A6A9B/file/D62C78201C2CCDEC0061FF770612F7F975F25896F1F7 (accessed May 18, 2022).

Grunér, M., M. Nordberg, and K. Lönnroth. 2022. Problems associated with mass border testing of COVID-19. *Scandinavian Journal of Public Health* 50(1):22-25. https://doi.org/10.1177/14034948211023659.

Gwee, S. X. W., P. E. Y. Chua, M. X. Wang, and J. Pang. 2021. Impact of travel ban implementation on COVID-19 spread in Singapore, Taiwan, Hong Kong and South Korea during the early phase of the pandemic: A comparative study. *BMC Infectious Diseases* 21(1):799. https://doi.org/10.1186/s12879-021-06449-1.

Hollingsworth, T. D., N. M. Ferguson, and R. M. Anderson. 2006. Will travel restrictions control the international spread of pandemic influenza? *Nature Medicine* 12(5):497-499. https://doi.org/10.1038/nm0506-497.

Jernigan, D. 2020. Update: Public health response to the coronavirus disease 2019 outbreak—United States, February 24, 2020. *MMWR: Morbidity and Mortality Weeky Report* 69(8):216-219.

Kim, C., K. Buckley, K. J. Marienau, W. L. Jackson, M. Escobedo, T. R. Bell, F. Alvarado-Ramy, and N. Marano. 2012. Public health interventions involving travelers with tuberculosis—U.S. ports of entry, 2007–2012. *MMWR: Morbidity and Mortality Weekly Report* 61(30):570-573. https://www.cdc.gov/mmwr/preview/mmwrhtml/mm6130a2.htm?s_cid=mm6130a2_w (accessed May 18, 2022).

Kraemer, M. U. G., C. H. Yang, B. Gutierrez, C. H. Wu, B. Klein, D. M. Pigott, L. du Plessis, N. R. Faria, R. Li, W. P. Hanage, J. S. Brownstein, M. Layan, A. Vespignani, H. Tian, C. Dye, O. G. Pybus, and S. V. Scarpino. 2020. The effect of human mobility and control measures on the COVID-19 epidemic in China. *Science* 368(6490):493-497. https://doi.org/10.1126/science.abb4218.

Kwok, W. C., C. K. Wong, T. F. Ma, K. W. Ho, L. W. Fan, K. F. Chan, S. S. Chan, T. C. Tam, and P. L. Ho. 2021. Modelling the impact of travel restrictions on COVID-19 cases in Hong Kong in early 2020. *BMC Public Health* 21(1):1878. https://doi.org/10.1186/s12889-021-11889-0.

Lai, S., N. W. Ruktanonchai, L. Zhou, O. Prosper, W. Luo, J. R. Floyd, A. Wesolowski, M. Santillana, C. Zhang, X. Du, H. Yu, and A. J. Tatem. 2020. Effect of non-pharmaceutical interventions to contain COVID-19 in China. *Nature* 585(7825):410-413. https://doi.org/10.1038/s41586-020-2293-x.

Lu, J., L. du Plessis, Z. Liu, V. Hill, M. Kang, H. Lin, J. Sun, S. François, M. U. G. Kraemer, N. R. Faria, J. T. McCrone, J. Peng, Q. Xiong, R. Yuan, L. Zeng, P. Zhou, C. Liang, L. Yi, J. Liu, J. Xiao, J. Hu, T. Liu, W. Ma, W. Li, J. Su, H. Zheng, B. Peng, S. Fang, W. Su, K. Li, R. Sun, R. Bai, X. Tang, M. Liang, J. Quick, T. Song, A. Rambaut, N. Loman, J. Raghwani, O. G. Pybus, and C. Ke. 2020. Genomic epidemiology of SARS-CoV-2 in Guangdong Province, China. *Cell* 181(5):997-1003.e1009.

Ma, Q., J. Liu, Q. Liu, L. Kang, R. Liu, W. Jing, Y. Wu, and M. Liu. 2021. Global percentage of asymptomatic SARS-CoV-2 infections among the tested population and individuals with confirmed COVID-19 diagnosis: A systematic review and meta-analysis. *JAMA Network Open* 4(12):e2137257. https://doi.org/10.1001/jamanetworkopen.2021.37257.

Martinez, L., K. Thomas, and J. Figueroa. 2010. Guidance from WHO on the prevention and control of TB during air travel. *Travel Medicine and Infectious Disease* 8(2):84-89. https://doi.org/10.1016/j.tmaid.2009.02.005.

Maskery, B. 2022. *CDC's Division of Global Migration and Quarantine: CDC.* Presentation to the National Academies of Sciences, Engineering, and Medicine Committee on Analysis to Enhance the Effectiveness of the Federal Quarantine Station Network.

Myers, J. F., R. E. Snyder, C. C. Porse, S. Tecle, P. Lowenthal, M. E. Danforth, E. Powers, A. Kamali, S. Jain, C. L. Fritz, and S. J. Chai. 2020. Identification and monitoring of international travelers during the initial phase of an outbreak of COVID-19—California, February 3–March 17, 2020. *MMWR: Morbidity and Mortality Weekly Report* 69(19):599-602. http://dx.doi.org/10.15585/mmwr.mm6919e4.

Nakazawa, E., H. Ino, and A. Akabayashi. 2020. Chronology of COVID-19 cases on the Diamond Princess cruise ship and ethical considerations: A report from Japan. *Disaster Medicine and Public Health Preparedness* 14(4):506-513. https://doi.org/10.1017/dmp.2020.50.

Niehus, R., P. M. De Salazar, A. R. Taylor, and M. Lipsitch. 2020. Using observational data to quantify bias of traveller-derived COVID-19 prevalence estimates in Wuhan, China. *The Lancet Infectious Diseases* 20(7):803-808. https://doi.org/10.1016/s1473-3099(20)30229-2.

Nuffield Council on Bioethics. 2020. *Ethical considerations in responding to the COVID-19 pandemic.* London, UK: Nuffield Council on Bioethics.

Ortega, L. S., R. B. Eidex, and M. S. Cetron. 2011. Migrant, immigrant, and refugee health. *Tropical Infectious Diseases: Principles, Pathogens and Practice* Jan:902-909.

Parino, F., L. Zino, M. Porfiri, and A. Rizzo. 2021. Modelling and predicting the effect of social distancing and travel restrictions on COVID-19 spreading. *Journal of the Royal Society Interface* 18(175):20200875. https://doi.org/10.1098/rsif.2020.0875.

Phares, C. R., Y. Liu, and Z. Wang. 2022. Disease surveillance among U.S.-bound immigrants and refugees—Electronic Disease Notification system, United States, 2014–2019. *MMWR: Morbidity and Mortality Weekly Report* 71(SS-2):1-21. http://dx.doi.org/10.15585/mmwr.ss7102a1.

Price, P. J. 2016. Quarantine and liability in the context of Ebola. *Public Health Reports* 131(3):500-503. https://dx.doi.org/10.1177/003335491613100316.

Rasicot, G. 2021. *DHS support to DGMQ: A collaborative approach.* Department of Homeland Security. Presentation to the National Acadmies of Sciences, Engineering, and Medicine Committee on Analysis to Enhance the Effectiveness of the Federal Quarantine Station Network.

Rispens, J. R., A. Freeland, B. Wittry, A. Kramer, L. Barclay, J. Vinjé, A. Treffiletti, and K. Houston. 2020. Notes from the field: Multiple cruise ship outbreaks of norovirus associated with frozen fruits and berries—United States, 2019. *MMWR: Morbidity and Mortality Weekly Report 2020* 69(16):501-502. http://dx.doi.org/10.15585/mmwr.mm6916a3.

Ronksley, P., T. Scory, R. Weaver, M. Lunney, R. Rodin, and M. Tonelli. 2021. The impact of vaccination status on importation of COVID-19 among international travellers. *Canada Communicable Disease Report* 47(11):473-475. https://doi.org/10.14745/ccdr.v47i11a05.

Rothstein, M. 2015. From SARS to Ebola: Legal and ethical considerations for modern quarantine. *Indiana Health Law Review* 12(1):227-280. https://doi.org/10.18060/18963.

Russell, T. W., J. T. Wu, S. Clifford, W. J. Edmunds, A. J. Kucharski, and M. Jit. 2021. Effect of internationally imported cases on internal spread of COVID-19: A mathematical modelling study. *Lancet Public Health* 6(1):e12-e20. https://doi.org/10.1016/S2468-2667(20)30263-2.

Salzer, H. J. F., E. Terhalle, and C. Lange. 2016. Extensively drug-resistant tuberculosis in long-term travellers. *The Lancet Infectious Diseases* 16(6):642-643. https://doi.org/10.1016/S1473-3099(16)30068-8.

Sell, T. K., M. P. Shearer, D. Meyer, M. Leinhos, E. Thomas, and E. G. Carbone. 2021. Public health implementation considerations for state-level Ebola monitoring and movement restrictions. *Disaster Medicine and Public Health Prepreparedness* 15(5):551-556. https://doi.org/10.1017/dmp.2020.45.

Stamatakis, C. E., M. E. Rice, F. M. Washburn, K. J. Krohn, M. Bannerman, and J. J. Regan. 2017. Maritime illness and death reporting and public health response, United States, 2010–2014. *Travel Medicine and Infectious Disease* 19:16-21. https://doi.org/10.1016/j.tmaid.2017.10.008.

U.S. Department of State. 2022. *COVID-19 travel information*. Bureau of Consular Affairs. https://travel.state.gov/content/travel/en/traveladvisories/covid-19-travel-information.html (accessed March 24, 2022).

USDA (U. S. Department of Agriculture). 2019. *Report on the importation of live dogs into the United States*. https://www.naiaonline.org/uploads/WhitePapers/USDA_DogImportReport6-25-2019.pdf.

Wells, C. R., P. Sah, S. M. Moghadas, A. Pandey, A. Shoukat, Y. Wang, Z. Wang, L. A. Meyers, B. H. Singer, and A. P. Galvani. 2020. Impact of international travel and border control measures on the global spread of the novel 2019 coronavirus outbreak. *Proceedings of the National Academy of Sciences of the United States of America* 117(13):7504-7509. https://dx.doi.org/10.1073/pnas.2002616117.

WHO (World Health Organization). 2016. *Guidance for managing ethical issues in infectious disease outbreaks*. Geneva, Switzerland: World Health Organization.

WHO. 2021. *WHO advice for international traffic in relation to the SARS-CoV-2 Omicron variant (b.1.1.529)*. https://www.who.int/news-room/articles-detail/who-advice-for-international-traffic-in-relation-to-the-sars-cov-2-omicron-variant (accesssed May 18, 2022).

4

New Technologies and Data Systems

The COVID-19 pandemic brought unprecedented challenges in disease detection and mitigation efforts due to the high volume and rapid spread of infections and insufficient public health resources with which to address them. These challenges exposed major gaps in national and global health capacities for early detection and swift response to an emerging pathogen of pandemic potential. Efforts to address these challenges resulted in advances in innovative technology for detecting, monitoring, and even predicting COVID-19. Among the many recent innovations in disease surveillance and control, this chapter focuses on those technologies that are relevant for the activities carried out by the Division of Global Migration and Quarantine (DGMQ). These include innovations for digital contact tracing, symptom reporting and monitoring, digital health certificates, digital data collection, data dashboards, and novel surveillance capabilities that have been developed and implemented at various scales and in different locations around the world since the outset of the COVID-19 pandemic.

In addition to highlighting some of these innovations and implementation examples, this chapter explores capabilities and concerns associated with novel digital data streams and collection. Although digital tracking and data collection can be more scalable, comprehensive, and expeditious than manual strategies, these technologies raise serious concerns regarding infringement on data privacy and pose ethical risks regarding personal and potentially sensitive data. This chapter considers the inherent tension between defending individual rights and liberties and protecting collective well-being. Ethics concerns associated with digital technologies for data collection and infectious disease control are explored in relation to the ethical considerations, such as protecting privacy, maintaining autonomy, promoting equity, minimizing risk of error, and ensuring accountability. Strategies to address ethical concerns while capitalizing on the benefits these technologies offer are discussed.

In addition to ethical considerations, the adoption of disease surveillance and monitoring technologies faces logistical challenges. Although incorporating digital technologies may allow the DGMQ to improve its capability to collect health data from travelers, trace transmission, and alert travelers of exposures, adoption depends on the public's trust and confidence in these interventions. Furthermore, data collection systems must be interoperable in order for the numerous stakeholders across various sectors to carry out their responsibilities in controlling major disease events. Key components needed to achieve interoperability of data systems are outlined. Opportunities for the DGMQ to leverage technology innovations hold potential to mitigate scale limitations of current screening and data collection processes to increase capacity to address a broad range of infection control purposes—including future pathogens of pandemic potential.

COVID-19 DETECTION TECHNOLOGIES

COVID-19 has resulted in numerous advances in technology, primarily in detection technology. Besides the gold standard of reverse transcriptase polymerase chain reaction (RT-PCR) in detecting COVID-19, new technologies have sought to improve on the limitations of RT-PCR, while keeping speed of detection a priority (Zhao et al., in press). These high-technology solutions are wide ranging—from other nucleic acid amplifications such as loop-mediated isothermal amplification (LAMP), serology-based assays, CRISPR-based assays, metagenomics next-generation sequencing (mNGS), aptamer-based assays, and lateral-flow technologies—to artificial intelligence- (AI-) assisted diagnoses, various spectroscopies including infrared spectroscopy, and nanotechnology-based approaches such as electrochemical sensors (Han et al., 2021; Li et al., 2020; Lukose et al., 2021). High-tech solutions tend to compensate along four dimensions, by providing (1) more information (e.g., miniaturized and multiplexed CRISPR [Zusi, 2020]), (2) more speed (e.g., field-effect transistor-based biosensors [Seo et al., 2020]), (3) more convenience (e.g., face masks with tiny, disposable sensors [Trafton, 2021], wearable device-detecting heart rate variability [Hirten et al., 2021]), or (4) more wide-ranging environmental methods of detection (e.g., detection of volatile organic compounds exhaled by positive cases [Giovannini et al., 2021], bioaerosol sensors). Beyond high-tech, additional nonintuitive and public-facing methods to detect, monitor, and even predict COVID-19 have emerged: sniffer dogs (Lippi et al., 2021), smartphone-app tracking (Verma and Mishra, 2020), and surveillance of sewage (CDC, 2022a;

Sweetapple et al., 2022). Future uses of these technologies include acting as tools to deal with future pandemics, especially as technologies such as the combined application of air collection and viral detection, whether it be polymerase chain reaction (PCR) analysis (BioFlyte, 2021) or cell analysis, will allow us to detect airborne disease of any kind in real time, decrease the spread/exposure early on, and formulate policies that pose the least interference to normal life. Outside COVID-19 and future pandemics, these advances also have the potential to assess populations' risks of exposure to infectious agents, through wastewater monitoring of infectious agents in a building or community, smartphone tracking for contact tracing, and crowd movement data for predicting outbreaks and hot spots (Zhao et al., in press). In addition, the role of AI–assisted radiologic computerized tomography (CT) scan (Harmon et al., 2020) and X-ray (Baltazar et al., 2021) readings developed during COVID-19 suggests that AI has supplemented, and will continue to supplement, our health decisions in the future.

USE OF INNOVATIVE AND INTEGRATIVE DIGITAL TECHNOLOGIES

Innovative digital technologies for collecting and aggregating data are essential tools for protecting the public's health from the introduction of diseases through international borders. During the COVID-19 pandemic, these types of technologies have been developed, refined, and implemented in countries around the world. The data collected using these technologies, as well as other novel data streams, can be used for a broad range of infection control purposes, including (1) contact tracing and proximity tracking to identify and monitor individuals potentially exposed to SARS-CoV-2 infection; (2) symptom reporting, monitoring, and tracking; (3) digital health certification, and (4) situational awareness and rapid epidemic intelligence. Coupled with advances in machine learning, AI, and other advanced analytical techniques for operationalizing the data, these new digital technologies and novel data streams provide public health authorities with a more powerful set of tools for surveillance and response than ever before. They also offer a range of opportunities for the DGMQ to leverage these innovative approaches to mitigate scale limitations of the current processes for implementing health screening and data collection at U.S. airports, as well as approaches to support health departments with post-arrival monitoring and follow-up of travelers.

Digital Technologies for Contact Tracing and Proximity Tracking

The World Health Organization (WHO) defines contact tracing as "the process of identifying, assessing, and managing people who have been exposed to a disease to prevent onward transmission" (WHO, 2020). When implemented systematically and comprehensively, contact tracing can contribute to the control of infectious disease outbreaks by breaking chains of transmission in a community through the identification and subsequent isolation and management of infectious individuals. However, successful contact tracing strategies must be bolstered by adequate health system capacity and resources to conduct contact investigations and then rapidly test, treat, and monitor potential cases (WHO, 2020).

Advantages of Digital Contact Tracing

Traditional manual contact tracing involves conducting interviews with people who are infected to identify other individuals with whom they have been in close-enough contact that the infection could potentially have been transmitted (Barrat et al., 2021). Identified contacts are then notified, generally by phone, that they may have been infected and are advised about appropriate measures, such as quarantine and symptom monitoring. This manual process has long been used as a public health strategy to help control the spread of infectious pathogens, but it is limited by its labor intensiveness, slowness, and reliance on the infected individual's recollection of their recent contacts (Barrat et al., 2021; Rodríguez et al., 2021). During the COVID-19 pandemic, the success of manual contact tracing efforts was undermined by a range of factors, including the volume of infections, insufficient public health resources and experienced contact tracing staff, lack of cooperation by contacts, and mistrust of government (Lo and Sim, 2021).

Digital contact tracing and proximity tracking technologies[1] can mitigate certain barriers to manual contact tracing by leveraging the ubiquity of data collected from smartphones to support efforts to control the spread of infectious diseases. As mobile phones have become an increasingly ubiquitous part of human lives, they are the most preferred implementation platform for digital contact tracing and tracking systems (Chowdhury et al., 2020). These applications are downloaded onto an individual's personal device and are used to determine whether that individual has come into contact with individual(s) who may by infected. The application then notifies the exposed individual and/or a public health agency with guidance about subsequent testing, treatment, isolation, monitoring, or other infection control measures (Ada Lovelace Institute, 2020).

---

[1] Although the two are often conflated, digital proximity tracking differs from digital contact tracing in that the latter is a newer approach to augment the former long-established public health practice. Proximity tracking involves the measurement of signal strength to ascertain whether two personal devices—typically smartphones, although wearable devices can also be tracked—have been in sufficiently close contact to risk the transmission of an infectious pathogen (WHO, 2020).

Digital contact tracing and proximity tracking applications can be used in several different ways to report cases of infection: (1) users can self-report infection through the application, with or without clinical or diagnostic confirmation, (2) a health care provider or test provider can report confirmed cases to the service operating the application, or (3) public health agencies or other authorities can input lists of individuals with confirmed infection (Ada Lovelace Institute, 2020). In addition, these digital technologies can be used to identify potentially infectious individuals with very large numbers of contacts, which could help to contain so-called "superspreader" events (Elmokashfi et al., 2021).

Digital contact tracing and tracking can be more scalable, comprehensive, and expeditious than manual strategies alone (Barrat et al., 2021; Grekousis and Liu, 2021). Although the superiority of digital contact tracing and tracking alone over traditional manual strategies has yet to be clearly established, digital solutions can complement and expedite manual strategies, particularly in the context of an accelerating outbreak (Anglemyer et al., 2020; Barrat et al., 2021; Elmokashfi et al., 2021; Ferretti et al., 2020; Grekousis and Liu, 2021). The scalability and speed of these technologies could be particularly advantageous for infection control efforts conducted by the DGMQ at borders and ports of entry, given the potential for large numbers of travelers quickly dispersing to different locations (Ferretti et al., 2020). It is also important to note that the use of these technologies is reliant on individuals' willingness to give permission for notifications.

Proximity and Location Awareness Technologies

Digital tracing and proximity tracking technologies rely on various types of device-based proximity and location awareness technologies that can be used to monitor individuals' movement, location, and proximity to other devices (see Table 4-1) (Grekousis and Liu, 2021). Location awareness technology is designed to indicate the precise location of a user—e.g., global navigation satellite systems (GNSS) or global positioning system (GPS). Technology such as WiFi (including the Encounter-Based Architecture for Contact Tracing [ENACT] and WifiTrace), Bluetooth Low Energy (BLE), Beacons, and Quick Response (QR) codes typically collect data only regarding devices' proximity to each other, although in some cases they can be used to detect a user's precise location as well (Grekousis and Liu, 2021).

Other technologies that can be leveraged for location and proximity tracking for public health purposes include cellular networks used by mobile phone providers, radio-frequency identification (RFID)—a wireless communication modality that utilizes radio frequency—and near-field com-

TABLE 4-1 Proximity and Location Awareness Technologies Used in Digital Contact Tracing and Tracking

Technology	LOCATION/PROXIMITY ACCURACY		COVID-19 TRACING		Privacy Concerns
	Outdoors	Indoors	Suitable for	Unsuitable for	
GNSS	10 m GPS only, 5 m GPS + WiFi	Most likely not operating	Outdoors/tracking overlapping routes/detection of hot spots	Indoors	High
BLE	< 2 m	< 2 m	Tracing individuals within 2 meters	Spaces with airborne transmission of SARS-CoV-2	Low to moderate
Beacons	Building level	Room/floor level	Same room/floor/building	Assessing the distance between individuals	Low to moderate
QR	Building level	Room/floor level	Same room/floor/building	Assessing the distance between individuals	Moderate to high
WiFi	Depending on Access Points	< 1 m	Indoors	Outdoors	Low to moderate
WB	Depending on UWB transmitters	< 0.5 m	Indoors	Currently, few smartphones have this technology	Low to moderate

NOTE: WB, wideband; UWB, ultra-wideband.
SOURCE: Data from Grekousis and Liu, 2021.

munication (NFC), which is applied in smart technologies such as access control systems and wireless payment and ticketing systems. Each technology has technical limitations in detecting distance in different scenarios, but most contact tracing system developers prefer BLE as the proximity sensing technology due to its cost-effectiveness, as BLE functionality is already built into smart devices by manufacturers (Min-Allah et al., 2021). Beyond case and contact identification, proximity and location awareness technologies on personal smartphones, as well as cameras, can also be used for monitoring individuals during isolation or following up with individuals who have traveled to settings with high risk of infectious disease transmission (Mbunge, 2020).

Comparing Centralized and Decentralized Architectures for Digital Data Management

Digital contact tracing and proximity tracking technologies can be distinguished by whether they use a centralized or decentralized system architecture to manage and share the collected data (Russo et al., 2021). A centralized system comprises a top-down architecture whereby data collected from smartphones or other peripheral devices are consolidated and stored in a central remote server, where the data are analyzed to inform public health actions (Grekousis and Liu, 2021; Russo et al., 2021). Decentralized systems utilize a bottom-up architecture in which data collected are retained and managed by the smartphones themselves, through technological infrastructure developed and provided by third-party companies, such as Apple or Google (Russo et al., 2021). The decentralized approach empowers individual users to control their own data and determine whether the data are uploaded to a central server (Grekousis and Liu, 2021). The centralized approach has the advantage of being able to collect greater volumes of data, but gives rise to serious concerns around the infringement on data privacy; the decentralized approach is less prone to privacy invasion, but may not be able to collect sufficient data for effective contact tracing and tracking unless an adequate number of users consent to share their data with the central repository (Grekousis and Liu, 2021).

Examples of Digital Contact Tracing and Tracking Technologies during the COVID-19 Pandemic

During the COVID-19 pandemic, multiple countries worldwide introduced digital contact tracing and proximity tracking using mobile devices to support efforts to curb the transmission of SARS-CoV-2. During the early phase of the pandemic, South Korea (Whitelaw et al., 2020), China (Golinelli et al., 2020), Taiwan (Golinelli et al., 2020), and Singapore (Savona, 2020) deployed digital contact tracing and tracking technologies that—in combination with strict transmission control measures, such as lockdowns and quarantine—appeared to contribute to limiting the spread of infection relatively successfully at the outset. As the pandemic continued through 2020 and 2021, many other countries also rolled out smartphone-based digital contact tracing applications. In Norway, for example, the introduction of a nationwide contact tracing application was found to have a tracing efficacy of 80 percent, with an estimated 11 percent of close contacts identified through digital tracing that could not have been identified via manual tracing (Elmokashfi et al., 2021).

A review of the use of COVID-19 contact tracing applications in nine countries found that they had variable and generally limited success in terms of public uptake and effectiveness in controlling transmission of SARS-CoV-2 in their populations (Russo et al., 2021). In the implementation of the National Health Service (NHS) COVID-19 app in England and Wales, it was found that for every percentage point increase in app use, there was a decrease in number of cases by 0.8 percent (Wymant et al., 2021). Additionally, based on the analysis and use of the SwissCOVID app in Switzerland, the digital contact tracing app was as effective as classic contact tracing (Salathe et al., 2020). However, subsequent reviews have suggested that if certain barriers related to ensuring data privacy, increasing effectiveness, encouraging population uptake, and addressing technical limitations are surmounted—discussed later in this chapter—the implementation of digital contact tracing and tracking efforts can be an effective component within a suite of public health infection control measures (Elmokashfi et al., 2021; Grekousis and Liu, 2021).

Digital Technologies for Symptom Reporting and Monitoring

During the COVID-19 pandemic, a number of countries have implemented digital systems and technologies for symptom reporting and monitoring. Symptom reporting and monitoring applications can be accessed on a website or installed on a personal smart device. Users can input details about their symptoms and, if they choose to do so, other personal information including demographics, geographic location, medical history, household information, and so forth (Ada Lovelace Institute, 2020). Data collected regarding individuals' symptoms can be used by public health authorities, for individuals that chose to do so, to support case identification and to initiate the processes of testing, treatment, and isolation of index patients and their contacts as appropriate.

The use of smart wearable technology—in conjunction with AI—is also emerging as a cost-effective strategy for screening, triaging, and remotely monitoring patients' symptoms and vital signs, such as blood pressure, electrocardiography (ECG), heart rate, and fever (Channa et al., 2021). Symptom checkers such as digital "smart" thermometers can be used to collect, analyze, and share health data, especially body temperature. Remote symptom monitoring via wearables is of particular value in settings where people have limited physical access to health care facilities, scenarios in which health care facilities are overwhelmed beyond capacity, and/or settings where the risk of infectious disease transmission is high in facilities (Channa et al., 2021; Mbunge, 2020). Moreover, symptom data can be used to understand disease transmission patterns and bolster epidemiological surveillance efforts as part of early warning systems, discussed in the next section.

Although the use of digital technologies for symptom reporting and monitoring, including wearables, is relatively new, it holds great promise in supporting the response to infectious disease outbreaks. Wearable digital technologies are associated with relatively fewer privacy risks than digital contact tracing and tracking, the data collected still need to be appropriately and robustly protected, particularly if they are collected in a centralized system (Ada Lovelace Institute, 2020). Other limitations include risks related to the quality of data collected (e.g., self-reported symptoms, false reporting), need to ensure linkages to care once symptoms detected, the impact of the digital divide in excluding vulnerable populations and worsening inequities, the need for more research to validate their efficacy and clinical utility, and the lengthy processes involved in gaining regulatory approval for medical devices (Ada Lovelace Institute, 2020; Channa et al., 2021).

Digital Health Certificates

Digital health certification is another application of novel digital health technology that emerged during the COVID-19 pandemic. Like data collected via other digital health technologies, digital health certification can be housed within a centralized system—such as electronic health records, health information systems, or public health authority databases—or a decentralized system, such as a physical record or digital token on an individual smart phone.

A number of countries have considered or implemented digital immunity certificates, a specific type of digital health certificate, to authenticate that a person has either already been infected with SARS-CoV-2 or has some other putative form of immunity against COVID-19 disease, such as vaccination (Ada Lovelace Institute, 2020). Generally, the aim of digital immunity certification is to ensure that a person can safely return to work, school, or other social settings. However, there is not yet a scientifically robust and empirically well-established way to establish that an individual has immunity against SARS-CoV-2 infection. Thus, the use of digital immunity certificates has garnered criticism and lack of support in some countries, such as the United Kingdom, due to the risk of negative societal consequences—for example, undermining of personal rights and freedoms, discrimination, and stigmatization (Ada Lovelace Institute, 2020). Additionally, the use of digital health certificates will require a standardization of health data collected and utilized by all institutions (Marios Angelopoulos et al., 2020). Further in this chapter, we discuss the importance of interoperability and the ethical consideration to ensure protection of patient information and rights.

Barriers to and Supports for the Use of Digital Technologies

Although innovative digital contact tracing and tracking technologies can serve as powerful mechanisms for collecting data to support the response to an infectious disease outbreak, epidemic, or pandemic, there are a range of technical and logistical barriers associated with their deployment in a population. Major technical barriers of interoperability and standardization are discussed in detail in the next section. Other technical limitations include digital technologies' imprecision in consistently and accurately detecting distance,[2] the ambiguity in defining what constitutes a "contact" at risk of transmitting or acquiring for a given infectious pathogen, inability to detect and trace contacts of asymptomatic patients, the potential for smartphone location or proximity technology to be deactivated or inaccurate, the need for skilled expertise to implement and maintain the system, the need to integrate complex security algorithms to ensure data protection and guard against fraud and abuse, and lack of supporting information and communication technology infrastructure and electronic health policy (Ada Lovelace Institute, 2020; Mbunge, 2020).

The use of digital contact tracing and tracking technologies are also associated with multiple ethics risks and legal challenges to individuals and societies, because the applications have access to individuals' personal and potentially sensitive data pertaining to their health behaviors, household location, traveling history, and other private information (Mbunge, 2020). A cross-country comparison of digital contact tracing apps used during the COVID-19 pandemic found that their success was limited due to concerns about data privacy (Russo et al., 2021). Another cross-country survey on the user acceptability of contact tracing apps deployed in France, Germany, Italy, the United Kingdom, and the United States reported that the main barriers to uptake were concerns about cybersecurity, privacy infringement, and lack of trust in the government (Altmann et al., 2020).

A fundamental logistical challenge in successfully deploying digital technologies for public health purposes is the need for a sufficiently widespread population uptake. For instance, some modeling studies have estimated that a digital proximity tracking technology would need to be adopted by 60–75 percent of a country's population to be maximally effective for contact identification during the COVID-19 pandemic (WHO, 2020). Other reviews have suggested that the uptake rate would need to

---

[2] Proximity of digital devices serves as the proxy for contact, but it depends upon measurable vectors (e.g., distance, time) that are inevitably imprecise to determine "contact"; this runs the risk of both false positives and false negatives. Additionally, is difficult for digital contact tracing to control for variables that underpin manual contact tracing (e.g., environment, ventilation, wind direction) (Ada Lovelace Institute, 2020).

reach at least 90 percent to control the epidemic if digital contact tracing is deployed in the absence of manual tracing (Grekousis and Liu, 2021). Digital and manual contact tracing are best used as complementary approaches to increase their overall effectiveness (Wang, 2021). However, widespread population uptake requires public trust and confidence that (1) the technology is effective in reducing the transmission of infectious disease and (2) the use of the technology does not compromise privacy, autonomy, or any other human rights and liberties (Ada Lovelace Institute, 2020; Nuffield Council on Bioethics, 2020; *The Lancet Digital Health*, 2020; WHO, 2020). Issues related to data security, privacy, ethics, equity, and autonomy—along with strategies to mitigate them—are discussed further later in this chapter.

Building trust and confidence in the technologies' effectiveness to encourage uptake is a reciprocal undertaking, because "…evidence of effectiveness directly affects uptake, while uptake directly affects effectiveness" (*The Lancet Digital Health*, 2020). Moreover, rolling out an untested and ultimately ineffective digital technology the first time can irrevocably undermine public trust in future interventions (Ada Lovelace Institute, 2020). Thus, an effective strategy for building public trust would involve a gradual process of robust research about the effectiveness of a new technology—and the minimum rate of population uptake required—that is coupled with clear and transparent communication to the public about its effectiveness, as well as its associated risks and uncertainties (Ada Lovelace Institute, 2020; Grekousis and Liu, 2021; *The Lancet Digital Health*, 2020).

Opportunities for the DGMQ to Leverage Innovative Digital Technologies

The DGMQ has the opportunity to incorporate and improve on the use of these novel digital technologies to gather health data from travelers, trace transmission, and alert exposures to travelers. This would also contribute to the development of scalable approaches to disease control strategies for large numbers of incoming travelers at borders and ports of entry. However, the successful use of these digital technologies is contingent on their integration within a strong network of supportive process and services for testing, treatment, and follow-up of people who have been or may have been exposed to infection. Success also depends on the public's trust and confidence in these interventions, as previously discussed. Thus, the DGMQ needs to consider strategies to engender public trust in the rollout and implementation of these technologies. The DGMQ is positioned to collaborate with other divisions within the U.S. Centers for Disease Control and Prevention (CDC) to lead conversations with stakeholders and local public health departments around innovative health technologies in order to increase public trust and lower barriers to uptake.

LEVERAGING NOVEL DIGITAL DATA STREAMS TO IMPROVE SITUATIONAL AWARENESS

To be of actionable value, data gleaned and aggregated from innovative digital technologies and novel digital data streams must be integrated into existing public health surveillance systems to detect outbreaks as early as possible and inform the appropriate response efforts to halt transmission. These surveillance systems often rely on natural language processing and machine learning to process, filter, analyze, and operationalize the enormous amount of data now available through these novel digital technologies and data sources (Allam et al., 2020; Jose et al., 2021). These new surveillance techniques could be leveraged by the DGMQ to improve its readiness and develop more flexible and targeted strategies for the control of infectious diseases at borders and ports of entry to the United States.

Novel Digital Data Streams

To support detection, monitoring, and public health decision making during an outbreak, these novel streams of data can be used to improve situational awareness at the early stage of a disease outbreak and to evaluate the risk of introduction of new pathogens through data dashboards, models, simulations, and other novel surveillance approaches to bolster rapid epidemic intelligence. In addition to those described in the previous section, other novel digital data streams that are increasingly being leveraged for public health surveillance of infectious diseases include online news websites, news aggregation services, internet search queries, video surveillance, participatory web platforms for self-reporting symptoms, and other streams of open-source and crowdsourced data (Aiello et al., 2020; Mello and Wang, 2020). Geospatial temporal data gleaned from smartphone geographic information system (GIS) functionality represent a vast and rich novel source of data about users' location and movements, which far exceeds the information that can be captured about geospatial and temporal patterns of infectious disease transmission using traditional surveillance methods (Hswen et al., 2022). The web-based application COVIDseeker, for example, captures and processes continuous fine-grained geospatial temporal data from smartphones to elucidate transmission of COVID-19 (Hswen et al., 2022).

In the context of an infectious disease outbreak, social media can serve as a powerful tool to disseminate public health information; data from social media platforms have also been used to help detect and predict cases of infectious diseases, such as influenza and malaria, prior to the COVID-19 pandemic (Tsao et al., 2021). During the COVID-19 pandemic, data from social media platforms were harnessed in a range of new ways for public health purposes. For example, the COVID-19 Surveiller[3] system was developed, using novel deep-learning models, to utilize social media users as "social sensors" for predicting pandemic trends—including new cases and death rates—as well as identifying potential risk factors to inform public health interventions (Jiang et al., 2022).

Innovations in Surveillance, Outbreak Analytics, and Early Warning Systems

The COVID-19 pandemic exposed major gaps in national and global health systems' capacities for early detection and swift response to an emerging pathogen of epidemic or pandemic potential. This has underscored the need for more effective early warning systems, given that epidemic and pandemic events are likely to become more frequent due to expanding urbanization, increasing global interconnectedness through travel and trade, the effects of climate change, and pervasive socioeconomic inequities (Carroll et al., 2021). As mentioned in Chapter 3, the CDC has established the new Center for Forecasting and Outbreak Analytics, which will bring together next-generation public health data, expert disease modelers, public health emergency responders, and high-quality communications to meet the needs of decision makers.

Early warning systems and other core capacities for surveillance can be strengthened by leveraging—in an effective and ethical way—the wealth of information that can be gleaned from novel data streams to augment traditional surveillance strategies. Early warning systems can be bolstered by rapid epidemic intelligence, which mines open-source data in tandem with traditional surveillance methods to detect early epidemic signals. Machine learning, AI, and algorithms for clinical diseases and syndromes are used to establish the baseline against which abnormal signals can be detected (Allam et al., 2020; Kogan et al., 2021). For example, at the outset of the COVID-19 pandemic, epidemiologists in China and Indonesia used data from the EpiWatch open-source observatory to detect early signals of pneumonia or severe acute respiratory illnesses as a proxy for COVID-19 (Kpozehouen et al., 2020; Thamtono et al., 2021). Computational approaches have been used to provide real-time risk assessment of case importation and their origin by leveraging on human mobility data. In particular, modeling and data analytics have been used to provide importation risk and estimates of the volume of imported cases during emerging health threats such as Ebola, Zika, and COVID-19 (Bogoch et al., 2015, 2016; Pullano et al., 2020).

---

[3] COVID-19 Surveiller is available at http://scaiweb.cs.ucla.edu/COVIDsurveiller (accessed February 22, 2022).

Other innovations in surveillance—leveraging novel digital data streams developed, refined, and implemented during the COVID-19 pandemic—include data dashboards, crowdsourcing, nowcasting, forecasting, and wastewater analysis. Early warning systems based on novel digital data sources, AI, and modeling approaches can provide real-time situational awareness and risk analysis.

Data Dashboards

During an outbreak, the synthesis of diverse data streams within broadly accessible online data dashboards can be powerful and dynamic tools for monitoring a rapidly evolving event, communicating epidemiological information, and informing decision making at all levels (Ivankovi et al., 2021). A data dashboard has been defined as a "visual representation of the most critical information required to fulfill one or more objectives, condensed on a single screen so that it can be monitored and understood at a glance" (Zhao et al., 2021). Using these dashboards, data can be represented in a range of visual formats including lists, tables, graphs, and maps.

Multiple dashboards were developed during the COVID-19 pandemic, as well as previous major infectious disease outbreaks, providing a range of critical information for monitoring and response. These dashboards include features such as (1) real- or near-real-time maps of cases and deaths, (2) predictive risk maps based on population geospatial mobility data, (3) maps of superspreader trajectories and contacts, (4) vaccine-related information, and (5) reactions to the evolving pandemic on social media platforms (Kamel Boulos and Geraghty, 2020; Zhao et al., 2021). For instance, Canada's Global Public Health Intelligence Network (GPHIN),[4] part of WHO's Global Outbreak Alert and Response Network (GOARN), was developed in 1997 and now monitors internet media from around the world to help detect potential infectious disease threats (Carter et al., 2020). In the United States, all 50 states developed their own publicly accessible dashboards for tracking and responding to the COVID-19 pandemic, albeit with significant variation in their design, content, and functions due to the lack of guidance for harmonization (Fareed et al., 2021). Other key examples of dashboards that leverage novel data streams to support rapid epidemic intelligence and the dissemination of information include:

---

[4] More information about the Global Public Health Intelligence Network is available from https://gphin.canada.ca/cepr/aboutgphin-rmispenbref.jsp?language=en_CA (accessed February 22, 2022).

- Johns Hopkins University's Center for Systems Science and Engineering (JHU CSSE) dashboard[5] (Kamel Boulos and Geraghty, 2020)
- A WHO Coronavirus (COVID-19) Dashboard[6] (Kamel Boulos and Geraghty, 2020)
- United States' HealthMap[7] (Kamel Boulos and Geraghty, 2020)
- Epidemic Intelligence from Open Sources (EIOS)[8]
- The International Society for Infectious Diseases' Program for Monitoring Emerging Diseases (ProMED)[9]

Crowdsourcing Surveillance

Innovations implemented during the COVID-19 pandemic demonstrated the value of crowdsourcing surveillance efforts in strengthening situational awareness, even before digital tracing and tracking applications or symptom reporting platforms were made available. In the early stages of an outbreak, compiling line lists of persons with suspected, probable, and confirmed infection—based on the evolving case definitions, in the case of a novel pathogen like SARS-CoV-2—is critical for initial assessment of the potential for epidemic growth and spread, as well as determining the appropriate infection control measures such as isolation and quarantine (Leung and Leung, 2020).

A crowdsourced surveillance approach was implemented in China in January 2020, when researchers aggregated daily case counts reported at the province level with individual-level data about patients with COVID-19 drawn from a Chinese social media network used by health care providers (Sun et al., 2020). This synthesized crowdsourced line list was consistent with the official national epidemiological reports provided by the Chinese government. In Japan, a crowdsourced data stream strengthened the national COVID-19 surveillance system, called "COvid-19: Operation for Personalized Empowerment to Render smart prevention And care seeking" (COOPERA). The system, which was implemented by a popular mobile messenger app used by the majority of the Japanese population, collected

---

[5] Johns Hopkins University's Center for Systems Science and Engineering dashboard is available at https://coronavirus.jhu.edu/data (accessed February 22, 2022).

[6] The WHO Coronavirus (COVID-19) Dashboard is available at https://COVID19.who.int (accessed February 22, 2022).

[7] HealthMap is available at https://www.healthmap.org/en (accessed February 22, 2022).

[8] The Epidemic Intelligence from Open Sources platform is available at https://www.who.int/initiatives/eios (accessed February 22, 2022).

[9] The International Society for Infectious Diseases' Program for Monitoring Emerging Diseases is available at https://promedmail.org/about-promed (accessed February 22, 2022).

information about users' COVID-19–like symptoms. Strong correlations between clusters of self-reported symptoms and outbreaks of confirmed cases highlighted crowdsourced data's value as an early warning system for impending outbreaks (Desjardins, 2020). In the United States, *Outbreaks Near Me* uses crowdsourced data to help individuals and public health agencies map the recent pandemic coronavirus, COVID-19, and the annual influenza (*Outbreaks Near Me*, 2022). This crowdsourced approach relies on voluntary participation from the general public that is asked to report their health status. Anybody can actively participate, providing weekly updates on their health status, even if no symptoms are experienced, and the data are used to provide a real-time awareness for the disease spread and prevalence. Similar approaches have been developed in Europe, Australia, and New Zealand (*FluTracking*, 2022; *GrippeCOVIDnet*, 2022).

Nowcasting and Forecasting

Timeliness is critical in detecting and responding appropriately to contain an infectious disease outbreak, but there are multiple points of potential delay from the point of symptom onset through care seeking, testing, and eventual reporting to public health authorities (Greene et al., 2021). Another innovation in epidemiological surveillance spurred by the COVID-19 pandemic is epidemic "nowcasting"—or "predicting the present"—to enhance situational awareness and inform response efforts during a rapidly evolving outbreak or epidemic by synthesizing real- or near-real-time data from novel data streams (Greene et al., 2021; Wu et al., 2021). One approach to nowcasting is to monitor prediagnostic streams of data—such as self-reported symptoms on participatory crowdsourced platforms and data from wearables and smart thermometers, internet searches, and social media posts—to gain a timely understanding of an evolving outbreak, albeit with a lack of specificity in distinguishing diseases such as SARS-CoV-2 from other respiratory illnesses with similar symptoms (Greene et al., 2021). A more specific approach is to draw upon partially reported disease data (e.g., near-real-time Google Trends data) and, accounting for reporting delays, using statistical methods and modeling to estimate cases and deaths that have not yet been reported (Greene et al., 2021). During the early months of the COVID-19 pandemic, the New York City Department of Health and Mental Hygiene effectively used nowcasting to support monitoring of reportable COVID-19 disease data (Greene et al., 2021). Modeling and artificial intelligence approaches are also used to generate insight into infectious disease outbreaks either through short-term forecasts or longer-term scenario analysis that assumes specific interventions or policies, such as in the specific CDC COVID-19 Forecasting Initiative (Allam, 2020, Biggerstaff et al., 2022). Advanced analytics have been used to anticipate the locations where the COVID-19 pandemic was expanding, estimate the international dissemination of cases, forecast the variation in time of the sources of new introductions of infections, and as well as for estimating the effect of border and travel restrictions policies (Bogoch et al., 2020; Chinazzi et al., 2020; Russell et al., 2021; Wells et al., 2020).

Wastewater Surveillance

Innovations in the use of wastewater as a novel data source for epidemiological surveillance were catalyzed by the discovery of SARS-CoV-2 in infected patients' feces and wastewater during the COVID-19 pandemic (Polo et al., 2020). This approach, which involves near-source tracking of sewage drains, municipal wastewater, sludge, and other sources to detect individual cases or small clusters of cases (Hassard et al., 2021; Philo et al., 2021), holds promise for facilitating early detection of infectious disease transmission dynamics, particularly in scenarios with limited testing and diagnostic reporting capacities (Peccia et al., 2020). Current research shows the utility of wastewater surveillance in static populations such as hospitals, prisons, and schools, and it could be beneficial for migrating populations if implemented in ports of entry, planes, cruise ships, or other modes of transportation (Hassard et al., 2021). The DGMQ should consider any forthcoming research on wastewater surveillance in migrating populations.

Opportunities for the DGMQ to Adopt or Leverage Surveillance Innovations

To enable detection of signals of outbreaks, the DGMQ could leverage these novel digital data sources and surveillance innovations to develop early warning systems that are integrated into border control. Data dashboards, developed extensively in the pandemic, could be adapted and expanded for the purposes of (1) collating real-time public health data, (2) keeping the public informed about an event as it evolves, and (3) supporting the clear and transparent communication of border policies.

INTEROPERABILITY OF DATA SYSTEMS

To effectively control a major infectious disease event by breaking the chains of transmission, a broad range of individuals, businesses, and institutions require up-to-date public health information about the epidemiology of the outbreak. These stakeholders span multiple sectors, including patients and their families, the health care sector (e.g., providers, administrators, laboratory staff, facility staff), public health authorities at the national level (e.g., the CDC) as well as at the state, tribal, local, and territorial levels, the transportation industry (e.g., airlines, cruise lines, other forms of public transport), and federal border control agencies. In the absence of efficient and harmonized channels of communication, critical information remains siloed within those various domains (Huang et al., in press).

To build a strong and effective health care and public health system capable of flexing to respond to a public health emergency, such as an infectious disease outbreak of pandemic potential, interoperability is an essential feature across channels of communication and other platforms for information exchange. Interoperability, which can be broadly defined[10] as the ability of two or more systems to exchange and utilize information, is the foundation of effective communications between data systems. Interoperability requires harmonization and standardization across all facets of digital systems, including data, content, platform, protocols, and downstream services (Savona, 2020). Issues that can impede interoperability include heterogeneous networking standards and communication protocols, differences in data semantics and ontology, nonstandardized data formats and structure, and diverse operating systems and programming languages, among others. It will be important for data formats and structure to be standardized across all platforms to avoid missing or redundant data, and to improve data quality (Mbunge, 2020).

Ideally, various digital contact tracing and tracking applications, regardless of their respective platforms, would be interoperable and easily integrated into health information systems to allow for rapid exchange of critical and timely information (Mbunge, 2020). However, these applications are generally developed independently using different protocols, data formats, and application programming interfaces (described in the following), thus are not necessarily interoperable (Mbunge, 2020). Interoperability is also essential for building public trust and confidence in the use of digital technologies for contact tracing and surveillance: "[i]nteroperability is widely considered as contributing to a transparent, trustworthy environment for citizens who face the choice of opting into a contact (or symptom, or immunity) tracing app, across devices, and countries" (Savona, 2020).

---

[10] The joint technical committee (JTC) of the International Organization for Standardization (ISO) and the International Electrotechnical Commission (IEC) defines interoperability as "the capability to communicate, execute programs, or transfer data among various functional units in a manner that requires the user to have little or no knowledge of the unique characteristics of those units" (ISO/IEC 2382-01 in Noura et al., 2018). The Institute of Electrical and Electronics Engineers (IEEE) defines the concept as the "ability of two or more systems or components to exchange information and to use the information that has been exchanged" (Noura et al., 2018).

Key Components of Interoperable Information Systems

Investments in data system interoperability can be lifesaving during a pandemic, but they can also improve day-to-day care coordination and reduce administrative costs in the U.S. health system (Carroll, 2020). Key components of interoperable health systems capable of timely, accurate, and comprehensive information exchange include application programming interfaces, data exchange platforms, electronic case reporting systems, and electronic laboratory reporting systems.

Application Programming Interfaces

At the core of interoperability are application programming interfaces (APIs). APIs serve as communication channels between databases, allowing for the electronic exchange of information. In order for two systems to communicate through an API, they must utilize a shared data standard. This shared data standard is similar to a language that two individuals can use to speak to one another. If the API supports the data standard that the two systems can read, it can be used for the exchange of information.

Data Exchange Platforms

During an infectious disease crisis, the ability to share data on clinical outcomes from electronic health record (EHR) patient registries seamlessly and efficiently through interoperable EHR system health care could contribute to strengthening response efforts both across and within health care systems (Jose et al., 2021). Data exchange networks have been developed to allow for the secure and rapid cross-organizational and vendor-neutral exchange of patient health information. One such data exchange network that has seen considerable success is Commonwell,[11] which was developed jointly by several health IT companies and launched in 2013. Currently, more than 25,000 providers have joined Commonwell and have received over 2 billion health records in total using the platform (CommonWell Health Alliance, n.d.). This platform enables the exchange of consolidated-clinical document architecture (C-CDA) documents. C-CDA is a data standard that enables the sharing of patient information such as encounters and clinical narratives between provider EHRs, regardless of vendor. By joining Commonwell, health care providers need not rely on dated technology, such as fax, to share patient medical records, allowing them to coordinate patient care more easily.

---

[11] More information about Commonwell is available from https://www.commonwellalliance.org (accessed February 22, 2022).

As different types of data—including mobile health and genomic data—become more widely available, C-CDA standards are being gradually replaced by the "fast healthcare interoperability resources" (FHIR) standard.[12] FHIR utilizes data elements, or "resources," that can be linked to other resources called references. Together, resources and their references make up data covering a wide range of health care scenarios. For instance, a resource such as "patient" can be linked to a reference such as "diagnosis" in order to store data about a patient's diagnosis by his or her health care provider. Health care APIs that use FHIR allow mobile or web-based applications to extract data from EHRs. Finally, to help facilitate electronic exchanges, the U.S. Department of Health and Human Services (HHS) recently released the first version of the Trusted Exchange Framework and Common Agreement (TEFCA) as a common set of guidelines for health information networks (HINs) (HealthIT, 2022).

Electronic Case Reporting

Timely, accurate, and efficient communication between health care providers and public health authorities is also of utmost importance during a pandemic. To report cases of infectious disease, health care providers can utilize a system called electronic case reporting (eCR), which facilitates the automated, real-time exchange of case report information from EHRs to public health agencies. Typically, eCR is not built into EHR systems, so health care providers may need to first integrate their EHR with the eCR Now FHIR App before they are able to use eCR.[13] The EHR then needs to be linked with the appropriate public health agency that receives the reports. The eCR system runs in the background of EHR systems, recognizing relevant information that must be reported and automatically sending that information to the appropriate public health agency via the Association of Public Health Laboratories (APHL) Informatics Messaging Services (AIMS) data exchange platform.[14] Once a public health agency receives a report, it conducts a review and analysis, and can make appropriate decisions to determine the necessary public health interventions.

As of November 12, 2021, more than 9,600 health care facilities have acquired eCR functionality. To encourage even more widespread use of eCR, the Centers for Medicare & Medicaid Services (CMS) Promoting Interoperability Program has included eCR in its criteria starting January 1,

---

[12] More information about the Fast Healthcare Interoperability Resources standard is available from https://www.altexsoft.com/blog/fhir-standard (accessed February 22, 2022).

[13] More information about the eCR Now FHIR App is available from https://ecr.aimsplatform.org/ecr-now-fhir-app (accessed February 22, 2022).

[14] More information about the Association of Public Health Laboratories (APHL) Informatics Messaging Services (AIMS) data exchange platform is available from https://www.aphl.org/programs/informatics/pages/aims_platform.aspx (accessed February 22, 2022).

2022.[15] The success of eCR implementation has the potential to drastically improve case reporting during a pandemic, allowing public health officials to quickly respond to outbreaks in communities through public health action such as contact tracing and quarantine. However, according to the 2018 American Hospital Association Annual Survey and IT Supplement, 41.2 percent of respondent hospitals reported that they had issues sending electronic data to public health agencies because these agencies could not receive the data. Some states had the majority of hospitals reporting this capability issue; only one state had zero hospitals reporting this problem (Holmgren et al., 2020). This highlights the need for the federal government to invest in public health IT infrastructure in a way commensurate to its investment in health care IT infrastructure.

Currently, the CDC's Data Modernization Initiative includes plans to integrate nationwide standards for data access and exchange that includes eCR (CDC, 2021a). This modernization of data systems was fueled by the COVID-19 pandemic but can be beneficial for broad disease surveillance (CDC, 2021a).

Electronic Laboratory Reporting

Data exchange between laboratories and public health agencies utilizes a system called electronic laboratory reporting (ELR). The ELR system is critical in ensuring efficient communication with public health agencies so that they can follow up with individuals with COVID-19 and carry out informed public health actions. Similar to eCR, ELR reports are sent to public health agencies through the AIMS platform using the HL7 v2.5.1 data standard.[16] Laboratory reports for SARS-CoV-2 are first sent to state and local public health agencies. This report contains identifying information about the patient, such as name and date of birth, that can aid state and local public health agencies in following up with the patient for contact tracing or other public health action. Before it is sent to the CDC, the ELR data are deidentified by removing information that could be used to determine the patient's identity (HHS, 2021).

Electronic Passenger Reporting

The CDC works with airlines and U.S. Customs and Border Protection (CBP) to collect passenger contact information to support aircraft contact investigations by state, tribal, local, and territorial public health partners.

---

[15] More information about the inclusion of electronic case records in CMS's Promoting Interoperability Program is available from https://www.cms.gov/Regulations-and-Guidance/Legislation/EHRIncentivePrograms (accessed February 22, 2022).

[16] More information about the HL7 v2.5.1 data standard is available from https://www.hl7.org/implement/standards/product_brief.cfm?product_id=98 (accessed February 22, 2022).

These investigations enable public health responses to inform exposed passengers, facilitate contact tracing to reduce the risk of subsequent disease transmission from disease exposures on commercial aircraft, and inform estimates of disease transmission risk on aircrafts. Aircraft contact investigations are typically initiated after the CDC receives a report from a health department or foreign ministry of health of a communicable disease case in a person with recent travel on a commercial aircraft. A Quarantine Station or headquarters staff member enters these reports into the Quarantine Activity Reporting System (QARS) and consults with medical officers and Quarantine Branch Aviation Activity staff to determine whether the case meets CDC criteria to initiate a contact investigation. If criteria for initiating a contact investigation are met, the CDC requests passenger manifest information from the airline for the passengers seated around the individual(s) reported to have had a communicable disease on board. The CDC uses disease-specific protocols that establish the exposure zone around an infectious passenger. A manifest is a document that contains the names, U.S. address for noncitizens or permanent residents, date of birth, gender, country of citizenship, and travel document type of individuals aboard the flight and assigned seat numbers on the flight. The airline manifest request timeline can be lengthy and the CDC may need to incorporate data from various formats used by different airlines. Additionally, accompanying contact information provided by airlines with manifests are frequently incomplete or incorrect. Airlines currently must also send passenger and crew manifests to CBP before departure to the United States; however, airlines are only required to transmit the name, date of birth, and gender for U.S. citizens and legal permanent residents. This process is primarily used to confirm the identities of travelers for national security purposes. CBP receives the manifests through the Advance Passenger Information System (APIS), which is an electronic data interchange system, and the airline submits the report through the APIS (or eAPIS[17]) portals (CBP, 2014). Additional contact information may be included from CBP's Automated Targeting System (ATS), which has the capacity to automatically generate a comprehensive record containing important information regarding the at-risk passengers on board the flight. To improve the quality of available traveler contact information, the CDC issued an order to require airlines to collect and maintain contact information, which became effective in November 2021 (*Federal Register*, 2021). Airlines have the option to share this information through their preestablished mechanism with the U.S. Department of Homeland Security (DHS) (e.g., APIS, eAPIS, or PNRGOV), through which the CDC can access data elements for public health contact investigations, or directly with the CDC on request.

---

[17] eAPIS is a web-based system that is available for use by smaller carriers. https://www.cbp.gov/travel/travel-industry-personnel/apis/eapis-transmission-system.

Cruise Ship Enhanced Data Collection

From April 2020 to January 15, 2022, all cruise ships operating or intending to operate in U.S. waters were required to submit the "Enhanced Data Collection (EDC) during COVID-19 Pandemic Form" daily (HHS and CDC, 2021). Upon the expiration of the Temporary Extension and Modification of Framework for Conditional Sailing Order (CSO) on January 15, 2022, the CDC implemented a voluntary COVID-19 risk mitigation program for cruise ships operating in U.S. waters that have chosen to participate in the CDC's COVID-19 Program for Cruise Ships (CDC, 2022b). As of May 2022, the CDC continues to require daily submission of the "Enhanced Data Collection (EDC) during COVID-19 Pandemic Form." If a cruise ship opts out of the program, then it is required to use the Maritime Conveyance Illness or the Death Investigation Form to report individual cases of COVID-19 and is asked to submit the Maritime Conveyance Cumulative Influenza/Influenza-Like Illness (ILI) Form (CDC, 2021b).

Efforts to Increase Interoperability

Over the past decade, the United States has made considerable progress in pushing forth efforts to increase interoperability. According to the 2019 National Electronic Health Records Survey, conducted prior to the COVID-19 pandemic, 89.9 percent of respondent physicians were using EHRs (CDC, 2019). In addition, 72.3 percent were using certified EHRs (CEHRs) that are eligible to receive financial benefits from the Medicare/Medicaid Promoting Interoperability Program based on adherence to EHR standards and program criteria. However, fax machines and email used in individual offices continue to be a significant portion of health information exchange, despite the wide adoption of EHRs. Fax machines are paper based and unreliable, often met with busy signals, and can run out of paper. Transmitting by email can also lead to delays—an important email sitting in an individual's inbox can also be easily missed or remain unread. Lack of interoperability between EHR systems and reliance on outdated and siloed technologies, such as email and fax, reduces the quality and efficiency of care coordination to successfully track, diagnose, and treat infectious diseases.

The Office of the National Coordinator for Health Information Technology (ONC), working with the CDC, has developed a framework to advance the health IT ecosystem for public health. On the top level, the TEFCA facilitates public health access to interoperability networks, which includes query capability to request records; core infrastructure to support exchange, including FHIR API; and consolidation of public health reporting over time. In the middle layer, clinical resources are among the health resources shared under the 21st Century Cures Act Final Rule of 2020, which prohibits information blocking when not sharing information (e.g., public health reporting data) as required by law. Finally, the fundamental point-to-point interoperability is supported by standard FHIR APIs, which allows push and pull of data in certified EHR systems with the additional ability to integrate decision support with passive triggers for important patient or public health events of interest.

Crowdsourcing Solutions to Interoperability Challenges

Like crowdsourcing epidemiological surveillance, crowdsourcing research and development of solutions to difficult technological challenges can be an effective strategy. "[H]arnessing the power of crowds and online communities […] can help tackle the COVID-19 pandemic, by providing original, actionable, quick, and low-cost solutions to the challenges of the current health and economic crisis" (Vermicelli et al., 2020, p. 183). For example, connectathons offer a powerful platform for crowdsourcing solutions to challenges related to interoperability. Connectathon events focus on developing an open, consensus-built interoperability specification that is both complete and demonstrates that it is possible for implementations written to that specification to connect with each other. Importantly, to encourage innovation, connectathons offer a safe venue for failure free of negative consequences of mistakes (Moehrke, 2013). Organizations such as Integrating the Healthcare Enterprise (IHE) convene these events regularly across the world (IHE, 2022). Box 4-1 provides more information on IHE Connectathons.

BOX 4-1
Connectathons of the Integrating the Healthcare Enterprise

The Integrating the Healthcare Enterprise describes its connectathons as follows:

> IHE Connectathons provide a detailed implementation and testing process to enable the adoption of standards-based interoperability by vendors and users of healthcare information systems. During a Connectathon systems exchange information with corresponding systems in a structured and supervised peer-to-peer testing environment, performing transactions required for the roles (IHE actors) they have selected to perform in carefully defined interoperability use cases (IHE profiles). Connectathons are held annually in Asia, Europe and North America. Thousands of vendor-to-vendor connections are tested each year. The results of testing are published in the Connectathon Results Database. The Connectathon provides detailed validation of the participants' interoperability and compliance with IHE profiles. Participating companies prepare for the event using testing software developed for this purpose. Connectathons offer vendors a unique opportunity for connectivity testing, removing barriers to integration that would otherwise often need to be addressed on site, at the customer's expense. Companies taking part have responded overwhelmingly that the IHE process addresses important issues in their product development plans.

SOURCE: https://www.ihe.net/participate/connectathon.

BALANCING ETHICAL RISKS WITH PUBLIC HEALTH BENEFITS

In considering whether to implement broad public health measures, there is an inherent tension between the need to defend individual rights and liberties and the responsibility to preserve the collective well-being. While the use of digital technologies to collect data for infectious disease control is a powerful tool for protecting public health, it also raises multiple ethical issues. Thus, deploying such measures inevitably requires a trade-off between the benefits of protecting the public's health and the potentially deleterious consequences for individuals. In the context of the COVID-19 pandemic, the use of digital technologies for measures like contact tracing, detection of individuals at risk of infection, quarantine enforcement, or epidemiological surveillance has sparked robust dialogue about how to ensure that these measures are taken in accordance with ethical principles.

Foundational Ethical Principles

The committee identified a set of foundational ethical principles that warrant close consideration by the DGMQ regarding the use of data collected via innovative digital technologies, novel data streams, and interoperative public health information systems for infection control measures. These principles include (1) protecting privacy, (2) maintaining autonomy, (3) promoting equity, (4) minimizing the risk of error, and (5) ensuring accountability.

Protecting Privacy

The nature of the data collected through these digital technologies makes it especially important to ensure data privacy and confidentiality, since there are multiple avenues for potential data misuse (e.g., governments targeting political opponents, use of data for migration policy enforcement) (Mello and Wang, 2020; WHO 2020). Given that concerns about privacy infringement and misuse of personal data pose major barriers to the implementation and uptake of infection control measures, the DGMQ needs to make every reasonable effort to protect data privacy and confidentiality.

Some of the privacy risks associated with data collected by public health authorities through these new digital technologies are similar to those associated with the huge volumes of personal data already collected by private companies on a large scale through their platforms, services, and products. For instance, some private companies are already aggregating and analyzing data collected by their own digital proximity tracking application—in some cases, they may even be doing so at the behest of public health agencies and sharing the data (WHO, 2020). However, there are some critical differences between the data use by public health authorities and that by private companies. For example, the former may require personal identifiers or take action based on the data received (Mello and Wang,

2020); the latter may not be aimed primarily at promoting collective public health, but instead driven by financial or other interests (Savona, 2020). Public perceptions about the use of personal data collected by public versus private entities also differ: "[w]hile accepting that their personal data are under the control of internet companies, most citizens seem unamenable to sharing their data for the public interest" (Russo et al., 2021).

Robust efforts to protect data privacy and confidentiality are critical for gaining public trust and encouraging uptake of public health measures. To engender trust, privacy protection can be incorporated into technological solutions—i.e., privacy by design—such that new developments ensure privacy protections by extracting data without sharing personal sensitive information (Nanni et al., 2021). For instance, the Decentralized Privacy-Preserving Proximity Tracing (DP-3T)[18] repository offers a secure, decentralized, privacy-preserving proximity tracing system that can support digitally enabled contact tracing while also providing the highest level of privacy protection and minimizing the data privacy and security risks to individuals (Ada Lovelace Institute, 2020).

Maintaining Autonomy

Respect for autonomy is a bioethics principle. Overriding the respect for autonomy should only be considered when the actions of the individual would seriously affect collective health (Dawson and Verweij, 2007). To adhere to the principle of respecting autonomy, the right of individuals to consent or right to refuse a public health measure should be preserved as far as possible when considering collective well-being. Through explicit and transparent practices to respect individual autonomy, the DGMQ can contribute to bolstering public trust and building "[…] a sense of collective interest in objectives that require individual commitment to be fully achieved" (Russo et al., 2021).

Individual autonomy can be undermined if the use of a digital data collection technology is made mandatory, if there are penalties for refusing to adopt it, or if appropriate informed consent policies are not in place (Savona, 2020). Informed consent policies should mitigate barriers related to language, accessibility, and health and technological literacy; they should also allow an individual to stop participating in data sharing at any time, despite the implications of individual withdrawals on the public health effectiveness of the broader contact tracing effort (Mbunge, 2020). User agreements can provide additional information and another layer of protection for users. With regard to digital contact tracing, informed consent is

---

[18] More information about the Decentralized Privacy-Preserving Proximity Tracing repository is available from https://github.com/DP-3T/documents (accessed February 22, 2022).

easier to obtain; however, for digital surveillance or digital fence it would require additional input from the public.

Not all digital data collection technologies currently in use allow people to decide whether to consent to their use (Mello and Wang, 2020), but there are others that require user consent before sending the data for central analysis (Wang, 2021). In a recent paper, Nanni et al. (2021) argue for a decentralized architecture for digital contact tracing, which could improve the autonomy of individuals. They also propose not to limit the data that the individual collects, but provide the individual with full control of that data—so the individual can decide what to share—through a "Personal Data Store" (Nanni et al., 2021). This contrasts with a centralized model for aggregating and analyzing digital contact tracing data used in China, based on the government's existing big data platform (Mao et al., 2021).

Promoting Equity

The DGMQ has an opportunity to reflect on how infection control measures informed by data collected through novel digital technologies and data steams can promote equity and avoid worsening existing inequities. Different social groups have varying degrees of access and capability to use digital technologies—that is, the "digital divide." For instance, use of applications for digital contact tracing often requires a smartphone, internet access, and technological acumen, which may exclude groups that are already vulnerable from participating in and realizing the benefits of digital contact tracing efforts (WHO, 2020). Moreover, overreliance on new digital modalities without the option to participate in traditional nondigital public health measures could further exacerbate existing health and socioeconomic inequities—for example, among older people who are not comfortable with smartphones or those who cannot afford them. Additionally, following the ethical principle of "ought implies can," those with access difficulties should never be penalized for lack of compliance with technology-based solutions. For example, it is unjust to penalize people, or place an undue burden on them without appropriate mechanisms for social support, whose socioeconomic conditions prevent them from self-isolating or complying with other public health measures based on digital contact tracing (*The Lancet Digital Health*, 2020).

Minimizing Risk of Error

Mistakes in identifying areas and individuals at high risk of infection could have negative public health and social consequences; thus, it is critical for the DGMQ to consider strategies to minimize the risk of error in the use of data collected via novel digital modalities (Mello and Wang, 2020).

Three factors—scope, speed, and sources—contribute to increasing the risk of such errors (Mello and Wang, 2020). Scope is an issue given the huge volumes of data that can be accrued through digital sources, because a relatively small percentage of errors in a dataset can parlay into a very large number of affected individuals. During an infectious disease emergency, the pressure to roll out digital technologies at high speed can undercut time needed for appropriate testing and evaluation, increasing the potential for errors in identifying individuals and communities at high risk; subsequent unnecessary public health measures, such as lockdowns, can have substantial social and economic consequences. Additionally, some sources of information in new digital datasets—for example, internet news sources, social media posts, self-reported symptoms—will inevitably be less reliable than traditional sources, which could contribute to the dissemination of misinformation (Mello and Wang, 2020). If digital technology is used, there should be systems of monitoring and correction in order to reduce burden of mistakes and bias in algorithms. Lastly, communities that are potentially impacted by mistakes in digital technologies should be a part of the decision process, so they are able to tolerate any consequences from mistakes and understand potential benefits of their use.

Ensuring Accountability

It is important to ensure that governments and private companies involved in the development and implementation of novel digital technologies are accountable for what they do with the data collected (Mello and Wang, 2020). In public health emergency situations, such as the COVID-19 pandemic, normally transparent democratic processes for ensuring accountability—which include opportunities for public discourse—may be temporarily overridden based on the need for rapid decision making and deployment of public health measures. This can lead to the development of technological solutions by small groups of public- and private-sector leaders operating outside of normal processes to ensure accountability (Mello and Wang, 2020).

Previous Recommendations to Mitigate Ethical Risks

As previously discussed, there are important ethical risks to be considered when designing and implementing digital technologies to collect and analyze large volumes of personal data for disease control. However, although " . . . these new uses of people's data can involve both personal and social harms . . . so does failing to harness the enormous power of data to arrest epidemics" (Mello and Wang, 2020, p. 952). In its deliberations, the committee considered the recommendations set forth by other groups who have also sought to strike the appropriate balance between mitigating these ethical risks and leveraging the full potential of data accrued through these new digital modalities. This section highlights previous recommendations for the use of digital technologies that the committee found helpful for its work.

Evaluate Proportionality

A common theme across previous recommendations is the need to evaluate and ensure the proportionality of public health interventions—particularly those that are novel and associated with ethical risks. This requires evaluating the burden, intrusiveness, and other risks posed by the measures with the potential for those measures to feasibly and effectively achieve their intended public health objectives (WHO, 2020). This assessment can guide decisions about whether the measure's effectiveness and impact require a trade-off relative to privacy protection that is proportional and commensurate to its public health benefits (WHO, 2020). According to the Nuffield Council on Bioethics,

> Any intervention should be proportionate to the effect that it is intended to achieve. Robust evidence that the intervention will be effective in achieving the desired aim is important in demonstrating that the intervention represents a proportionate response to the particular health threat. In the absence of such evidence, interventions held to be necessary should be accompanied by an evidence-gathering programme. The more intrusive the intervention, the stronger the justification and the clearer the evidence required. (Nuffield Council on Bioethics, 2020)

Similarly, a recommendation made in a review by the Ada Lovelace Institute maintains that assessments of necessity and proportionality should consider not only the effectiveness of an intervention in achieving its objective, but also whether the aim could be achieved by less intrusive measures (Ada Lovelace Institute, 2020). That is, more intrusive interventions are unlikely to be proportionate if there are less intrusive interventions available that are likely to be just as effective (Nuffield Council on Bioethics, 2020).

After assessing the risks of using a technology compared to the impact of choosing not to use it—for example, evaluating whether digitally enabled surveillance can help to avoid strict lockdown measures—the least burdensome and intrusive alternative should be chosen (Mello and Wang, 2020). Assessing the least restrictive and burdensome options may require both a global assessment across populations most likely to be affected and those most likely to experience severe hardship. If a technology proves to be insufficiently effective to warrant ethical risks, it should be phased out (WHO, 2020). The WHO also recommends that measures should be temporary, with data collected via digital technologies and sources being deleted after a certain period—and that privacy-preserving measures should be used in technology design (e.g., avoiding the use of geographic position tracking for digital proximity tracking) (WHO, 2020).

Maintaining Autonomy

Previous recommendations commonly hold that measures should be taken to maintain and improve individual autonomy. For example, the WHO maintains that governments should not mandate the use of digital technologies for public health purposes; instead, individuals should be empowered with the ability to make an informed and voluntary—to the extent possible—decision about whether to download and utilize those technologies (WHO, 2020). Given the lack of robust evidence for their effectiveness, mandating the use of digital contact tracing and tracking applications would contravene the principles of necessity and proportionality (Ada Lovelace Institute, 2020). Moreover, mandating their use would likely be unenforceable and undermine their effectiveness and uptake (Ada Lovelace Institute, 2020). The WHO further recommends against the provision of incentives or other inducements for individual use offered by public authorities or private entities, nor should individuals be denied benefits or services for refusal, discontinuation, or withdrawal of consent at any time. Additionally, individuals should have the autonomy to delete any personal data that have been collected or stored by the technology (WHO, 2020).

Protecting Privacy

Previous recommendations focus heavily on the critical need to protect the privacy and confidentiality of personal data collected via digital technologies and novel data streams (Ada Lovelace Institute, 2020; WHO, 2020). Many different measures can be taken to protect privacy, including the use of privacy-preserving data storage infrastructure, ensuring the security of data from various types of misuse, and retaining data for a minimal and limited period of time (WHO, 2020).

A major privacy-related issue to consider is the choice between using a centralized or decentralized architecture to store digital data (see previous section). Both approaches can potentially be privacy preserving, albeit with respective vulnerabilities that would have to be addressed. The WHO's guidance highlights an emerging consensus among data protection authorities toward decentralized approaches as the preferred option for protecting privacy (WHO, 2020). Within a decentralized structure, users have a greater degree of autonomy to grant or withdraw consent for their personal data to be shared with health authorities or other parties (WHO, 2020).

Regardless of the storage infrastructure used, it is also crucial that the appropriate data protection and privacy laws are in place and adhered to, ideally supported by regulations for legal and limited data processing, restrictions to prevent data misuse, oversight processes, and sunset clauses for discontinuing and dismantling technology after the emergency period has passed (WHO, 2020). The WHO guidance also recommends aggregating and anonymizing data collected (when possible), strictly limiting the retention of data to the emergency response period, and then subsequently deleting all data collected for those purposes (WHO, 2020).

Promoting Equity

Previous studies recommended that measures should be taken to promote equity and avoid exacerbating existing inequities (Ada Lovelace Institute, 2020; Nuffield Council on Bioethics, 2020; WHO, 2020). To that end, the WHO (2020) recommended that strategies should be designed specifically to reach marginalized populations and vulnerable communities. To improve access to technologies among people with limited resources, potential approaches include lowering mobile data costs for digital public health technologies and making certain types of smart devices more affordable and accessible (WHO, 2020). Another approach is to develop digital contact tracing applications based on unstructured supplementary service data (USSD), which does not require internet access, thus enabling people living in areas without internet access to participate in digitally enabled public health measures (Mbunge, 2020).

Minimizing Data and Restricting Use

The WHO's guidance strongly recommends implementing strategies to minimize the amount of personal data collected through digital modalities and to restrict data use to the extent possible (WHO, 2020). Specifically, the collection, retention, and processing of data should be limited in scope to the minimum amount necessary to achieve the intended public health objective. For digital proximity tracking, for example, data collection practices should not require users to disclose their identities, locations, or the specific timing of a proximity event (WHO, 2020). The WHO also calls for the strict prohibitions on the sale or use of collected data for any type of commercial purposes or the sharing of data with government entities or third parties that are not directly involved in the ongoing public health response, including law enforcement or immigration agencies (WHO, 2020).

Testing and Evaluation

The WHO recommends conducting careful testing and evaluation of novel technological solutions both before and after implementation, as most of these technologies currently lack a sound evidence base for their effectiveness across different settings and scenarios (WHO, 2020). Prior to widespread rollout of technologies, they should be robustly tested to ensure they are functionally effective, technically robust, and without security flaws. After implementation, it is critical to continuously evaluate and monitor the performance of the technology on the ground in real-world conditions. Ideally, an independent party would conduct the monitoring and evaluation, then publish and publicly disseminate the results (WHO, 2020).

Integrating the Use of Digital Data in Interventions

The use of digital data collection technologies—such as digital contact tracing and proximity tracking applications—should be situated within a broader set of public health interventions, practices, investments, and policies (WHO, 2020). Additionally, the WHO recommends that governments and health systems should carefully consider and clearly communicate to the public how the chosen suite of policies, interventions, and technologies integrate and complement each other within the broader strategy (WHO, 2020). Similarly, a review by the Ada Lovelace Institute maintains that these digital technologies can be effective as part of an emergency or transition strategy, but cautions that they are not a replacement for sound policy. Instead, "[t]echnologies must form a part of holistic public health surveillance strategies and other pandemic response initiatives; without supporting evidence, they can and should not replace other proven methods" (Ada Lovelace Institute, 2020, p. 9).

Ensuring Public Engagement, Transparent Accountability, and Strong Governance

Previous recommendations highlight the importance of ensuring robust public engagement, transparent accountability, and strong governance in implementing digital technologies for disease control (Ada Lovelace Institute, 2020; Mello and Wang, 2020; Nuffield Council on Bioethics, 2020; WHO, 2020).

"Effective policy interventions using technology take account of the social dimension of technology and its societal impact, are designed with the input and involvement of people across society, and are monitored and evaluated to assess their social impact on individuals and communities" (Ada Lovelace Institute, 2020, p.9). Thus, digital technologies should be implemented using a transparent process governed by independent oversight bodies that include members of the public (including representatives of marginalized groups), public health authorities, ethics experts, data and technology experts, and civil society organizations (Ada Lovelace Institute, 2020; Mello and Wang, 2020; WHO, 2020). In addition to being an ethical imperative, this type of participatory approach to oversight can also promote voluntary uptake and participation (WHO, 2020).

The DGMQ needs to design and implement clear, inclusive, and trustworthy public communication strategies to explain the rationale for implementing digital technologies for the common good, as well as providing justification for the collection and use of personal data (Nuffield Council on Bioethics, 2020; WHO, 2020). Data-processing agreements also need to disclose to users whether and why personal data may be shared with third parties (Ienca and Vayena, 2020). Ensuring accountability also requires appropriate safeguards against abuse, with individuals provided the opportunity to challenge data collection and use practices. Persons who are subject to unwarranted surveillance should have access to "effective remedies and mechanisms of contestation" (WHO, 2020).

CONCLUSIONS AND RECOMMENDATIONS

Conclusions

Conclusion 4-1: The DGMQ's data technology infrastructure is woefully inadequate to address modern disease threats in a context of rapid global travel, as evidenced by shortcomings of manpower and efficiency in addressing the COVID-19 pandemic. The continued reliance on manual data entry is reflective of this gap.

Conclusion 4-2: The use of innovative technologies—such as novel detection technology, digital data sources, early warning systems, and outbreak analytics—has a role in integrated border control. Data dashboards were developed extensively during the COVID-19 pandemic and could be extended to collate real-time public health data in order to keep the public informed and support the communication of border policies. The use of digital technologies to gather health data from travelers, trace transmission, and alert travelers to exposures is at the core of scalable systems for disease control at the border and in transportation. The success of any digital technology solution stems not only from the technology itself, but also from the process and services surrounding it. Successful technology implementation is also heavily dependent on the trust of the citizens. Therefore, efforts need to be in place to increase the trust level and thus the adoption rate of the technologies in society.

Conclusion 4-3: Interoperability across data systems is critical for maintaining up-to-date information on the spread of contagious diseases such as COVID-19, given the various parties—including health care providers, laboratory personnel, public health agencies, and border control agencies—who rely on this data to carry out their missions. As health information technology developers continue to increase functionality in mobile health applications and electronic health records, legislation on the proper use of information will likely be needed. Investments in data system interoperability can be life saving during a pandemic, would improve day-to-day care coordination, and could generate financial benefits to the United States.

Conclusion 4-4: The use of digital technologies, novel data streams, and interoperative public health information systems holds enormous potential for infectious disease control. However, multiple ethical issues are associated with these tools. The DGMQ will need to ensure that any and all use of innovative technologies follows a careful consideration of its ethical aspects, including concerns about autonomy, privacy, and equity. In order to achieve this, an improved process of governance needs to be established. This could take the form of an oversight structure, either embedded in the existing CDC ethics committee or as part of the activities of a new DGMQ advisory committee. Good governance also requires that the DGMQ effectively communicate to the public about the need to use these technologies and their role as part of a comprehensive set of interventions. Thus, this issue represents another area for improvement is strategic communications.

Conclusion 4-5: The framework of the Office of the National Coordinator for Health Information Technology (ONC) outlines a pathway to an interoperable health data ecosystem and can be used by health care institutions to modernize their data systems by fully utilizing health care interoperability concepts, such as data standards and application programming interfaces. Once institutions have established data connections, queries have to be performed to pick up real-time signals using various machines.

Recommendations

**Recommendation 4-1: The Division of Global Migration and Quarantine (DGMQ) should increase and improve the use of innovative technology to aid in outbreak detection and response and to mitigate disease transmission. The DGMQ should improve readiness and develop flexible and targeted strategies for disease control at the border. The DGMQ should incorporate and improve on the use of digital technologies to gather health data from travelers, trace transmission, and alert travelers to exposures. These practices will also allow the development of scalable approaches to disease control strategies for large numbers of incoming travelers.

Recommendation 4-2: The Division of Global Migration and Quarantine (DGMQ) should support the adoption of the Office of the National Coordinator for Health Information Technology (ONC) roadmap by health care and public health practitioners. The DGMQ should work with the ONC to facilitate the ONC roadmap and interoperability networks. Connectathons—events that allow providers, organizations, or other implementers to learn from developers, conduct testing, and practice exchanging data asynchronously across agencies—are an example of how this could occur. As health information technology developers continue to increase functionality in mobile health applications and electronic health records, the DGMQ should identify gaps and opportunities in legislation and regulation to support the proper use and transfer of information across data systems.

Recommendation 4-3: The Division of Global Migration and Quarantine (DGMQ) should ensure that all uses of digital technologies, novel data streams, and interoperative public health information systems follows a careful consideration of their ethical aspects and that all actions are in accordance with existing regulations for the protection of personal data. In order to achieve this, the DGMQ should put an oversight structure in place.

REFERENCES

Ada Lovelace Institute. 2020. *Exit through the app store? A rapid evidence review on the technical considerations and societal implications of using technology to transition from the COVID-19 crisis.* London, UK: Ada Lovelace Institute.

Aiello, A. E., A. Renson, and P. N. Zivich. 2020. Social media- and internet-based disease surveillance for public health. *Annual Review of Public Health* 41:101-118. https://dx.doi.org/10.1146/annurev-publhealth-040119-094402.

Allam, Z., G. Dey, and D. S. Jones. 2020. Artificial intelligence (AI) provided early detection of the coronavirus (COVID-19) in China and will influence future urban health policy internationally. *AI* 1(2):156-165. https://doi.org/10.3390/ai1020009.

Altmann, S., L. Milsom, H. Zillessen, R. Blasone, F. Gerdon, R. Bach, F. Kreuter, D. Nosenzo, S. Toussaert, and J. Abeler. 2020. Acceptability of app-based contact tracing for COVID-19: Cross-country survey study. *JMIR Mhealth Uhealth* 8(8):e19857. https://doi.org/10.2196/19857.

Anglemyer, A., T. H. Moore, L. Parker, T. Chambers, A. Grady, K. Chiu, M. Parry, M. Wilczynska, E. Flemyng, and L. Bero. 2020. Digital contact tracing technologies in epidemics: A rapid review. *Cochrane Database of Systematic Reviews* 8(8):CD013699. https://doi.org/10.1002/14651858.cd013699.

Baltazar, L. R., M. G. Manzanillo, J. Gaudillo, E. D. Viray, M. Domingo, B. Tiangco, and J. Albia. 2021. Artificial intelligence on COVID-19 pneumonia detection using chest xray images. *PLOS ONE* 16(10):e0257884. https://doi.org/10.1371/journal.pone.0257884.

Barrat, A., C. Cattuto, M. Kivela, S. Lehmann, and J. Saramaki. 2021. Effect of manual and digital contact tracing on COVID-19 outbreaks: A study on empirical contact data. *Journal of the Royal Society Interface* 18(178):20201000. https://doi.org/10.1098/rsif.2020.1000.

Biggerstaff, M., R. B. Slayton, M. A. Johansson, and J. C. Butler. 2022. Improving pandemic response: Employing mathematical modeling to confront coronavirus disease 2019. *Clinical Infectious Diseases* 74(5):913-917. https://doi.org/10.1093/cid/ciab673.

BioFlyte. 2021. *Bioflyte launches first field deployable airborne COVID-19 detection system to improve school and workplace safety.* https://bioflyte.com/2021/05/26/bioflyte-launches-first-field-deployable-airborne-COVID-19-detection-system-to-improve-school-and-workplace-safety (accessed February 23, 2022).

Bogoch, I. I., M. I. Creatore, M. S. Cetron, J. S. Brownstein, N. Pesik, J. Miniota, T. Tam, W. Hu, A. Nicolucci, S. Ahmed, J. W. Yoon, I. Berry, S. I. Hay, A. Anema, A. J. Tatem, D. MacFadden, M. German, and K. Khan. 2015. Assessment of the potential for international dissemination of Ebola virus via commercial air travel during the 2014 West African outbreak. *The Lancet* 385(9962):29-35. https://doi.org/10.1016/s0140-6736(14)61828-6.

Bogoch, I. I., O. J. Brady, M. U. G. Kraemer, M. German, M. I. Creatore, M. A. Kulkarni, J. S. Brownstein, S. R. Mekaru, S. I. Hay, E. Groot, A. Watts, and K. Khan. 2016. Anticipating the international spread of Zika virus from Brazil. *The Lancet* 387(10016):335-336. https://doi.org/10.1016/S0140-6736(16)00080-5.

Bogoch, I. I., A. Watts, A. Thomas-Bachli, C. Huber, M. U. Kraemer, and K. Khan. 2020. Potential for global spread of a novel coronavirus from China. *Journal of Travel Medicine* 27(2):taaa011. https://doi.org/10.1093/jtm/taaa011.

Carroll, D., S. Morzaria, S. Briand, C. K. Johnson, D. Morens, K. Sumption, O. Tomori, and S. Wacharphaueasadee. 2021. Preventing the next pandemic: The power of a global viral surveillance network. *BMJ* 372:n485. https://doi.org/10.1136/bmj.n485.

Carroll, L. 2020. More than a third of U.S. healthcare costs go to bureaucracy. *Reuters Health*. https://www.reuters.com/article/idUSKBN1Z5261 (accessed March 4, 2022).

Carter, D., M. Stojanovic, P. Hachey, K. Fournier, S. Rodier, Y. Wang, and B. de Bruijn. 2020. Global public health surveillance using media reports: Redesigning GPHIN. *Studies in Health Technology and Informatics* 270:843-847. https://doi.org/10.3233/SHTI200280.

CBP (U.S. Customs and Border Protection). 2014. *eAPIS Online Transmission System.* https://www.cbp.gov/travel/travel-industry-personnel/apis/eapis-transmission-system (accessed May 10, 2022).

CDC (Centers for Disease Control and Prevention). 2019. *National Electronic Health Records Survey public use file national weighted estimates.* Atlanta, GA: CDC National Center for Health Statistics. https://www.cdc.gov/nchs/data/nehrs/2019NEHRS-PUF-weighted-estimates-508.pdf (accessed May 19, 2022).

CDC. 2021a. *CDC's COVID-19 data improvement.* https://www.cdc.gov/coronavirus/2019-ncov/science/data-improvements.html (accessed March 4, 2022).

CDC. 2021b. *Cruise ships: Reporting maritime death or illness (non-gastrointestinal) to DGMQ.* https://www.cdc.gov/quarantine/cruise/reporting-deaths-illness/index.html (accessed March 15, 2022).

CDC. 2022a. *National wastewater surveillance system (NWSS)*. https://www.cdc.gov/healthywater/surveillance/wastewater-surveillance/wastewater-surveillance.html (accessed February 23, 2022).

CDC. 2022b. *Technical instructions for CDC's COVID-19 program for cruise ships operating in U.S. waters*. https://www.cdc.gov/quarantine/cruise/management/technical-instructions-for-cruise-ships.html (accessed May 10, 2022).

Channa, A., N. Popescu, J. Skibinska, and R. Burget. 2021. The rise of wearable devices during the COVID-19 pandemic: A systematic review. *Sensors* 21(17):5787. https://doi.org/10.3390/s21175787.

Chinazzi, M., J. T. Davis, M. Ajelli, C. Gioannini, M. Litvinova, S. Merler, Y. P. A. Pastore, K. Mu, L. Rossi, K. Sun, C. Viboud, X. Xiong, H. Yu, M. E. Halloran, I. M. Longini, Jr., and A. Vespignani. 2020. The effect of travel restrictions on the spread of the 2019 novel coronavirus (COVID-19) outbreak. *Science* 368(6489):395-400. https://dx.doi.org/10.1126/science.aba9757.

Chowdhury, M. J. M., M. S. Ferdous, K. Biswas, N. Chowdhury, and V. Muthukkumarasamy. 2020. COVID-19 contact tracing: Challenges and future directions. *IEEE Access* 8:225703-225729. doi:10.1109/ACCESS.2020.3036718.

CommonWell Health Alliance. n.d. *Frequently asked questions*. https://www.commonwellalliance.org/about/faq (accessed February 22, 2022).

Dawson, A., M. Verweij, and M. Verweij. 2007. *Ethics, prevention, and public health*. New York, NY: Oxford University Press on Demand.

Desjardins, M. R. 2020. Syndromic surveillance of COVID-19 using crowdsourced data. *The Lancet Regional Health Western Pacific* 4:100024. https://doi.org/10.1016/j.lanwpc.2020.100024.

Elmokashfi, A., J. Sundnes, A. Kvalbein, V. Naumova, S. A. Reinemo, P. M. Florvaag, H. K. Stensland, and O. Lysne. 2021. Nationwide rollout reveals efficacy of epidemic control through digital contact tracing. *Nature Communications* 12(1):5918. https://doi.org/10.1038/s41467-021-26144-8.

Fareed, N., C. M. Swoboda, S. Chen, E. Potter, D. T. Y. Wu, and C. J. Sieck. 2021. U.S. COVID-19 state government public dashboards: An expert review. *Applied Clinical Informatics* 12(2):208-221. https://doi.org/10.1055/s-0041-1723989.

Federal Register. 2021. *Temporary suspension of dogs entering the United States from high risk rabies countries*. https://www.govinfo.gov/content/pkg/FR-2021-06-16/pdf/2021-12418.pdf (accessed March 10, 2022).

Ferretti, L., C. Wymant, M. Kendall, L. Zhao, A. Nurtay, L. Abeler-Dörner, M. Parker, D. Bonsall, and C. Fraser. 2020. Quantifying SARS-CoV-2 transmission suggests epidemic control with digital contact tracing. *Science* 368(6491):eabb6936. https://doi.org/10.1126/science.abb6936.

FluTracking. 2022. https://info.flutracking.net (accessed March 10, 2022).

Giovannini, G., H. Haick, and D. Garoli. 2021. Detecting COVID-19 from breath: A game changer for a big challenge. *ACS Sensors* 6(4):1408-1417. https://doi.org/10.1021/acssensors.1c00312.

Golinelli, D., E. Boetto, G. Carullo, A. G. Nuzzolese, M. P. Landini, and M. P. Fantini. 2020. Adoption of digital technologies in health care during the COVID-19 pandemic: Systematic review of early scientific literature. *Journal Medical Internet Research* 22(11):e22280. https://doi.org/10.2196/22280.

Greene, S. K., S. F. McGough, G. M. Culp, L. E. Graf, M. Lipsitch, N. A. Menzies, and R. Kahn. 2021. Nowcasting for real-time COVID-19 tracking in New York City: An evaluation using reportable disease data from early in the pandemic. *JMIR Public Health and Surveillence* 7(1):e25538. https://doi.org/10.2196/25538.

Grekousis, G., and Y. Liu. 2021. Digital contact tracing, community uptake, and proximity awareness technology to fight COVID-19: A systematic review. *Sustainable Cities and Societies* 71:102995. https://doi.org/10.1016/j.scs.2021.102995.

GrippeCOVIDnet. 2022. https://www.grippenet.fr (accessed March 10, 2022).

Han, T., H. Cong, Y. Shen, and B. Yu. 2021. Recent advances in detection technologies for COVID-19. *Talanta* 233:122609. https://doi.org/10.1016/j.talanta.2021.122609.

Harmon, S. A., T. H. Sanford, S. Xu, E. B. Turkbey, H. Roth, Z. Xu, D. Yang, A. Myronenko, V. Anderson, and A. Amalou. 2020. Artificial intelligence for the detection of COVID-19 pneumonia on chest CT using multinational datasets. *Nature Communications* 11(1):4080. https://doi.org/10.1038/s41467-020-17971-2.

Hassard, F., L. Lundy, A. C. Singer, J. Grimsley, and M. Di Cesare. 2021. Innovation in wastewater near-source tracking for rapid identification of COVID-19 in schools. *The Lancet Microbe* 2(1):e4-e5. https://doi.org/10.1016/S2666-5247(20)30193-2.

HealthIT.gov. 2022. *Trusted Exchange Framework and Common Agreement (TEFCA)*. https://www.healthit.gov/topic/interoperability/trusted-exchange-framework-and-common-agreement-tefca (accessed February 26, 2022).

HHS (U.S. Department of Health and Human Services). 2021. *COVID-19 pandemic response, laboratory data reporting: CARES Act Section 18115*. Washington, DC: U.S. Department of Health and Human Services. https://www.hhs.gov/sites/default/files/COVID-19-laboratory-data-reporting-guidance.pdf (accessed February 14, 2022).

HHS and CDC. 2021. *Temporary extension & modification of framework for conditional sailing order (CSO) for cruise ships operating or intending to operate in U.S. waters*. https://www.federalregister.gov/documents/2021/10/28/2021-23573/temporary-extension-and-modification-of-framework-for-conditional-sailing-order-cso-for-cruise-ships (accessed February 14, 2022).

Hirten, R. P., M. Danieletto, L. Tomalin, K. H. Choi, M. Zweig, E. Golden, S. Kaur, D. Helmus, A. Biello, R. Pyzik, A. Charney, R. Miotto, B. S. Glicksberg, E. P. Bottinger, L. Keefer, M. Suarez-Farinas, G. N. Nadkarni, and Z. A. Fayad. 2021. Use of physiological data from a wearable device to identify SARS-CoV-2 infection and symptoms and predict COVID-19 diagnosis: Observational study. *Journal of Medical Internet Research* 23(2):e26107. https://preprints.jmir.org/preprint/26107.

Holmgren, A. J., N. C. Apathy, and J. Adler-Milstein. 2020. Barriers to hospital electronic public health reporting and implications for the COVID-19 pandemic. *Journal of the American Medicinal Informatics Association* 27(8):1306-1309. https://doi.org/10.1093/jamia/ocaa112.

Hswen, Y., E. Yom-Tov, V. Murti, N. Narsing, S. Prasad, G. W. Rutherford, and K. Bibbins-Domingo. 2022. COVIDseeker: A geospatial temporal surveillance tool. *International Journal of Environmental Research and Public Health* 19(3):1410. https://doi.org/10.3390/ijerph19031410.

Huang, J., N. R. Shah, and C. J. Wang. In press. Interoperability of healthcare and public health data: Key to future of pandemic preparedness.

Ienca, M., and E. Vayena. 2020. On the responsible use of digital data to tackle the COVID-19 pandemic. *Nature Medicine* 26(4):463-464. https://doi.org/10.1038/s41591-020-0832-5.

IHE International. 2022. *IHE Connectathon: A unique testing opportunity*. https://www.ihe.net/participate/connectathon (accessed May 15, 2022).

Ivanković, D., E. Barbazza, V. Bos, Ó. Brito Fernandes, K. Jamieson Gilmore, T. Jansen, P. Kara, N. Larrain, S. Lu, B. Meza-Torres, J. Mulyanto, M. Poldrugovac, A. Rotar, S. Wang, C. Willmington, Y. Yang, Z. Yelgezekova, S. Allin, N. Klazinga, and D. Kringos. 2021. Features constituting actionable COVID-19 dashboards: Descriptive assessment and expert appraisal of 158 public web-based COVID-19 dashboards. *Journal of Medical Internet Research* 23(2):e25682-e25682. https://doi.org/10.2196/25682.

Jiang, J. Y., Y. Zhou, X. Chen, Y. R. Jhou, L. Zhao, S. Liu, P. C. Yang, J. Ahmar, and W. Wang. 2022. COVID-19 Surveiller: Toward a robust and effective pandemic surveillance system based on social media mining. *Philosophical Transactions of the Royal Society A* 380(2214):20210125. https://doi.org/10.1098/rsta.2021.0125.

Jose, T., D. O. Warner, J. C. O'Horo, S. G. Peters, R. Chaudhry, M. J. Binnicker, and C. D. Burger. 2021. Digital health surveillance strategies for management of coronavirus disease 2019. *Mayo Clinical Proceedings: Innovations, Quality, and Outcomes* 5(1):109-117. https://doi.org/10.1016/j.mayocpiqo.2020.12.004.

Kamel Boulos, M. N., and E. M. Geraghty. 2020. Geographical tracking and mapping of coronavirus disease COVID-19/severe acute respiratory syndrome coronavirus 2 (SARS-CoV-2) epidemic and associated events around the world: How 21st century GIS technologies are supporting the global fight against outbreaks and epidemics. *International Journal of Health Geographics* 19(1):8. https://doi.org/10.1186/s12942-020-00202-8.

Kogan, N. E., L. Clemente, P. Liautaud, J. Kaashoek, N. B. Link, A. T. Nguyen, F. S. Lu, P. Huybers, B. Resch, and C. Havas. 2021. An early warning approach to monitor COVID-19 activity with multiple digital traces in near real time. *Science Advances* 7(10):eabd6989. https://doi.org/10.1126/sciadv.abd6989.

Kpozehouen, E. B., X. Chen, M. Zhu, and C. R. Macintyre. 2020. Using open-source intelligence to detect early signals of COVID-19 in China: Descriptive study. *JMIR Public Health and Surveillience* 6(3):e18939. https://doi.org/10.2196/18939.

Leung, G. M., and K. Leung. 2020. Crowdsourcing data to mitigate epidemics. *The Lancet Digital Health* 2(4):e156-e157. https://doi.org/10.1016/S2589-7500(20)30055-8.

Li, H. Y., W. N. Jia, X. Y. Li, L. Zhang, C. Liu, and J. Wu. 2020. Advances in detection of infectious agents by aptamer-based technologies. *Emerging Microbes & Infections* 9(1):1671-1681. https://doi.org/10.1080/22221751.2020.1792352.

Lippi, G., C. Mattiuzzi, and B. M. Henry. 2021. Are sniffer dogs a reliable approach for diagnosing SARS-CoV-2 infection? *Diagnosis* 8(4):446-449. https://doi.org/10.1515/dx-2021-0034.

Lo, B., and I. Sim. 2021. Ethical framework for assessing manual and digital contact tracing for COVID-19. *Annals of Internal Medicine* 174(3):395-400. https://doi.org/10.7326/M20-5834.

Lukose, J., S. Chidangil, and S. D. George. 2021. Optical technologies for the detection of viruses like COVID-19: Progress and prospects. *Biosensors and Bioelectronics* 178:113004. https://doi.org/10.1016/j.bios.2021.113004.

Mao, Z., H. Yao, Q. Zou, W. Zhang, and Y. Dong. 2021. Digital contact tracing based on a graph database algorithm for emergency management during the COVID-19 epidemic: Case study. *JMIR Mhealth Uhealth* 9(1):e26836. https://doi.org/10.2196/26836.

Marios Angelopoulos, C., A. Damianou, and V. Katos. 2020. DHP framework: Digital health passports using blockchain—use case on international tourism during the COVID-19 pandemic. arXiv: 2005.08922v2.

Mbunge, E. 2020. Integrating emerging technologies into COVID-19 contact tracing: Opportunities, challenges and pitfalls. *Diabetes & Metabolic Syndrome: Clinical Research & Reviews* 14(6):1631-1636. https://doi.org/10.1016/j.dsx.2020.08.029.

Mello, M. M., and C. J. Wang. 2020. Ethics and governance for digital disease surveillance. *Science* 368(6494):951-954. https://doi.org/10.1126/science.abb9045.

Min-Allah, N., B. A. Alahmed, E. M. Albreek, L. S. Alghamdi, D. A. Alawad, A. S. Alharbi, N. Al-Akkas, D. Musleh, and S. Alrashed. 2021. A survey of COVID-19 contact-tracing apps. *Computers in Biology and Medicine* 137:104787. https://doi.org/10.1016/j.compbiomed.2021.104787.

Moehrke, J. 2013. *What is connectathon? Healthcare Exchange Standards.* https://healthcare secprivacy.blogspot.com/2013/11/what-is-connectathon.html (accessed February 26, 2022).

Nanni, M., G. Andrienko, A. L. Barabasi, C. Boldrini, F. Bonchi, C. Cattuto, F. Chiaromonte, G. Comande, M. Conti, M. Cote, F. Dignum, V. Dignum, J. Domingo-Ferrer, P. Ferragina, F. Giannotti, R. Guidotti, D. Helbing, K. Kaski, J. Kertesz, S. Lehmann, B. Lepri, P. Lukowicz, S. Matwin, D. M. Jimenez, A. Monreale, K. Morik, N. Oliver, A. Passarella, A. Passerini, D. Pedreschi, A. Pentland, F. Pianesi, F. Pratesi, S. Rinzivillo, S. Ruggieri, A. Siebes, V. Torra, R. Trasarti, J. V. D. Hoven, and A. Vespignani. 2021. Give more data, awareness and control to individual citizens, and they will help COVID-19 containment. *Ethics and Information Technology* 23(1):1-6. https://doi.org/10.1007/s10676-020-09572-w.

Noura, M., M. Atiquzzaman, and M. Gaedke. 2018. Interoperability in internet of things: Taxonomies and open challenges. *Mobile Networks and Applications* 24(3):796-809. https://doi.org/10.1007/s11036-018-1089-9.

Nuffield Council on Bioethics. 2020. *Ethical considerations in responding to the COVID-19 pandemic.* London, UK: Nuffield Council on Bioethics.

Outbreaks Near Me. 2022. https://outbreaksnearme.org/us/en-U.S. (accessed March 10, 2022).

Peccia, J., A. Zulli, D. E. Brackney, N. D. Grubaugh, E. H. Kaplan, A. Casanovas-Massana, A. I. Ko, A. A. Malik, D. Wang, M. Wang, J. L. Warren, D. M. Weinberger, W. Arnold, and S. B. Omer. 2020. Measurement of SARS-CoV-2 RNA in wastewater tracks community infection dynamics. *Nature Biotechnology* 38(10):1164-1167. https://doi.org/10.1038/s41587-020-0684-z.

Philo, S. E., E. K. Keim, R. Swanstrom, A. Q. W. Ong, E. A. Burnor, A. L. Kossik, J. C. Harrison, B. A. Demeke, N. A. Zhou, N. K. Beck, J. H. Shirai, and J. S. Meschke. 2021. A comparison of SARS-CoV-2 wastewater concentration methods for environmental surveillance. *Science of the Total Environment* 760:144215. https://doi.org/10.1016/j.scitotenv.2020.144215.

Polo, D., M. Quintela-Baluja, A. Corbishley, D. L. Jones, A. C. Singer, D. W. Graham, and J. L. Romalde. 2020. Making waves: Wastewater-based epidemiology for COVID-19—approaches and challenges for surveillance and prediction. *Water Research* 186:116404. https://doi.org/10.1016/j.watres.2020.116404.

Pullano, G., F. Pinotti, E. Valdano, P.-Y. Boëlle, C. Poletto, and V. Colizza. 2020. Novel coronavirus (2019-nCoV) early-stage importation risk to Europe, January 2020. *Eurosurveillance* 25(4):2000057. https://doi.org/10.2807/1560-7917.ES.2020.25.4.2000057.

Rodríguez, P., S. Graña, E. E. Alvarez-León, M. Battaglini, F. J. Darias, M. A. Hernán, R. López, P. Llaneza, M. C. Martín, RadarCOVIDPilot Group, O. Ramirez-Rubio, A. Romaní, B. Suárez-Rodríguez, J. Sánchez-Monedero, A. Arenas, and L. Lacasa. 2021. A population-based controlled experiment assessing the epidemiological impact of digital contact tracing. *Nature Communications* 12(1):587. https://doi.org/10.1038/s41467-020-20817-6.

Russell, T. W., J. T. Wu, S. Clifford, W. J. Edmunds, A. J. Kucharski, and M. Jit. 2021. Effect of internationally imported cases on internal spread of COVID-19: A mathematical modelling study. *The Lancet Public Health* 6(1):e12-e20. https://doi.org/10.1016/s2468-2667(20)30263-2.

Russo, M., C. Ciccotti, F. De Alexandris, A. Gjinaj, G. Romaniello, A. Scatorchia, and G. Terranova. 2021. A cross-country comparison of contact-tracing apps during COVID-19. *VOXEU CEPR.*

Salathe, M., C. Althaus, N. Anderegg, D. Antonioli, T. Ballouz, E. Bugnon, S. Capkun, D. Jackson, S. I. Kim, J. Larus, N. Low, W. Lueks, D. Menges, C. Moullet, M. Payer, J. Riou, T. Stadler, C. Troncoso, E. Vayena, and V. von Wyl. 2020. Early evidence of effectiveness of digital contact tracing for SARS-CoV-2 in Switzerland. *Swiss Medical Weekly* 150:w20457. https://doi.org/10.4414/smw.2020.20457.

Savona, M. 2020. The saga of the COVID-19 contact tracing apps: Lessons for data governance. *SPRU Working Paper Series (SWPS)* 2020-10:1-12. https://ssrn.com/abstract=3645073.

Seo, G., G. Lee, M. J. Kim, S.-H. Baek, M. Choi, K. B. Ku, C.-S. Lee, S. Jun, D. Park, and H. G. Kim. 2020. Rapid detection of COVID-19 causative virus (SARS-CoV-2) in human nasopharyngeal swab specimens using field-effect transistor-based biosensor. *ACS Nano* 14(4):5135-5142.

Sun, K., J. Chen, and C. Viboud. 2020. Early epidemiological analysis of the coronavirus disease 2019 outbreak based on crowdsourced data: A population-level observational study. *Lancet Digital Health* 2(4):e201-e208. https://doi.org/10.1016/S2589-7500(20)30026-1.

Sweetapple, C., P. Melville-Shreeve, A. S. Chen, J. M. Grimsley, J. T. Bunce, W. Gaze, S. Fielding, and M. J. Wade. 2022. Building knowledge of university campus population dynamics to enhance near-to-source sewage surveillance for SARS-CoV-2 detection. *Science of the Total Environment* 806:150406. https://doi.org/10.1016/j.scitotenv.2021.150406.

Thamtono, Y., A. Moa, and C. R. MacIntyre. 2021. Using open-source intelligence to identify early signals of COVID-19 in Indonesia. *Western Pacific Surveillance and Response Journal* 12(1):40-45. https://doi.org/10.5365/wpsar.2020.11.2.010.

The Lancet Digital Health. 2020. Contact tracing: Digital health on the frontline [Editorial]. *The Lancet Digital Health* 2(11):e561. https://doi.org/10.1016/S2589-7500(20)30251-X.

Trafton, A. 2021. New face mask prototype can detect COVID-19 infection. *MIT News*. https://news.mit.edu/2021/face-mask-COVID-19-detection-0628 (accessed February 23, 2022).

Tsao, S. F., H. Chen, T. Tisseverasinghe, Y. Yang, L. Li, and Z. A. Butt. 2021. What social media told us in the time of COVID-19: A scoping review. *The Lancet Digital Health* 3(3):e175-e194. https://doi.org/10.1016/s2589-7500(20)30315-0.

Verma, J., and A. S. Mishra. 2020. COVID-19 infection: Disease detection and mobile technology. *PeerJ* 8:e10345. https://doi.org/10.7717/peerj.10345.

Vermicelli, S., L. Cricelli, and M. Grimaldi. 2020. How can crowdsourcing help tackle the COVID-19 pandemic? An explorative overview of innovative collaborative practices. *R&D Management* 51(2):183-194. https://doi.org/10.1111/radm.12443.

Wang, C. J. 2021. Contact-tracing app curbed the spread of COVID in England and Wales. *Nature* 594(7863):336-337.

Wells, C. R., P. Sah, S. M. Moghadas, A. Pandey, A. Shoukat, Y. Wang, Z. Wang, L. A. Meyers, B. H. Singer, and A. P. Galvani. 2020. Impact of international travel and border control measures on the global spread of the novel 2019 coronavirus outbreak. *Proceedings of the National Academy of Sciences of the United States of America* 117(13):7504-7509. https://doi.org/10.1073/pnas.2002616117.

Whitelaw, S., M. A. Mamas, E. Topol, and H. G. C. Van Spall. 2020. Applications of digital technology in COVID-19 pandemic planning and response. *The Lancet Digital Health* 2(8):e435-e440. https://doi.org/10.1016/s2589-7500(20)30142-4.

WHO (World Health Organization). 2020. *Ethical considerations to guide the use of digital proximity tracking technologies for COVID-19 contact tracing: Interim guidance, 28 May 2020*. Geneva, Switzerland: World Health Organization.

Wu, J. T., K. Leung, T. T. Y. Lam, M. Y. Ni, C. K. H. Wong, J. S. M. Peiris, and G. M. Leung. 2021. Nowcasting epidemics of novel pathogens: Lessons from COVID-19. *Nature Medicine* 27(3):388-395. https://doi.org/10.1038/s41591-021-01278-w.

Wymant, C., L. Ferretti, D. Tsallis, M. Charalambides, L. Abeler-Dorner, D. Bonsall, R. Hinch, M. Kendall, L. Milsom, M. Ayres, C. Holmes, M. Briers, and C. Fraser. 2021. The epidemiological impact of the NHS COVID-19 app. *Nature* 594(7863):408-412. https://doi.org/10.1038/s41586-021-03606-z.

Zhao, B., M. Kim, and E. W. Nam. 2021. Information disclosure contents of the COVID-19 data dashboard websites for South Korea, China, and Japan: A comparative study. *Healthcare* 9(11):1487. https://doi.org/10.3390/healthcare9111487.

Zhao, D., F.-S. W. Lee, and C. J. Wang. In press. COVID-19 detection technologies in pandemic control. *JAMA*.

Zusi, K. 2020, April 19. New technology could provide rapid detection of COVID-19. *The Harvard Gazette*. https://news.harvard.edu/gazette/story/2020/04/new-technology-could-provide-rapid-detection-of-covid-19 (accessed May 19, 2022).

5

Improving Coordination and Collaboration

The Centers for Disease Control and Prevention (CDC) Division of Global Migration and Quarantine (DGMQ) accomplishes its duties through a mixture of regulatory authorities as well as operating partnerships. Because of the nature of the quarantine function, these partnerships are with both domestic and international partners in government and the private sector—other nation's quarantine and disease control organizations; U.S. federal agencies; state, tribal, local and territorial (STLT) agencies; and private sector aviation and maritime industries. Any industry that moves people or goods is a potential partner of the DGMQ because of the disease control nature of their mission. Together, this constellation of partnerships serves as the organizational and operational framework for implementing policies and activities to prevent and control the onward transmission of communicable diseases. There is an opportunity to strengthen these working relationships to achieve better operational efficiencies and improve overall disease control efforts. By strengthening these working relations through predefined strategies, the DGMQ can improve accomplishing its core missions. As with all partnerships, the goal is achieving the mission while optimizing the outcomes for partners.

The COVID-19 pandemic has also revealed a wide range of partners with whom the CDC, and specifically the DGMQ, ought to have significant functional relationships. While some work is accomplished through the DGMQ's regulatory authority, most of the division's work is accomplished through working relationships with both governmental and predominantly nongovernmental partners. These relationships are best nurtured by regular formal engagement to solve problems and address issues before a serious emergency occurs, not in the midst of one. The pandemic has also revealed opportunities to strengthen relationships with STLT agencies as well as international and private industry partners. This chapter synthesizes approaches for improving coordination and collaboration among federal, state, local, and international partners and systems to protect communities across the United States from infectious disease threats.

COLLABORATION WITH KEY PARTNERS

Collaboration with Federal Interagency Partners

The CDC's DGMQ partners with a range of federal interagency partners—both within HHS and across other departments, including

- U.S. Department of Health and Human Services (HHS)
  o Office of the Assistant Secretary for Preparedness and Response (ASPR)
    o Office of Global Affairs (OGA)
    o Administration for Children and Families (ACF)
    o Office of Refugee Resettlement (ORR)
    o Food and Drug Administration (FDA)
- U.S. Department of Homeland Security (DHS)
  o Countering Weapons of Mass Destruction Office (CWMD)
  o U.S. Customs and Border Protection (CBP)
  o U.S. Coast Guard (USCG)
  o Transportation Security Administration (TSA)
  o U.S. Citizenship and Immigration Services (USCIS)
  o DHS/CBP-National Targeting Center (NTC)
  o Immigration and Customs Enforcement (ICE)
- U.S. Department of Defense (DoD)
- U.S. Department of Transportation (DOT)
  o Federal Aviation Administration (FAA)
  o Federal Transit Administration
  o Federal Railroad Administration
- U.S. Department of State (DOS)
  o Bureau of Population, Refugees, and Migration
  o Bureau of Consular Affairs
  o American Citizens Services and Crisis Management[1]
- Department of Justice (DOJ)
- U.S. Department of Agriculture (USDA)
  o Animal and Plant Health Inspection Service (APHIS)

---

[1] https://www.usa.gov/federal-agencies/american-citizens-services-and-crisis-management (accessed April 15, 2022).

IMPROVING COORDINATION AND COLLABORATION

- U.S. Department of the Interior (DOI)
  o U.S. Fish and Wildlife Service (FWS)

For example, Figure 5-1 shows the agencies involved in importation of animals at ports of entry.

Collaboration with the Department of Homeland Security

The missions of DHS and the DGMQ intersect in terms of protecting the public, safeguarding borders, enabling legitimate trade and travel, and providing services to immigrants, refugees, and travelers (see Figure 5-2). DHS and the CDC partnered in supporting the U.S. government response to COVID-19,[2] information sharing, and providing operational support to enhance screening and testing for COVID-19 and for Ebola during the 2014–2016, 2019, and 2021 outbreaks (Rasicot, 2021). DHS interagency coordination during the COVID-19 pandemic led to a number of international travel orders, including a mask mandate, vaccine order, global testing order, and contact data collection. Other interagency coordination efforts include the Runway to Recovery framework, which provides guidance to airports and airlines to mitigate the effects of COVID-19 on travel. Developed by DHS, DOT, and HHS,[3] Runway to Recovery includes steps

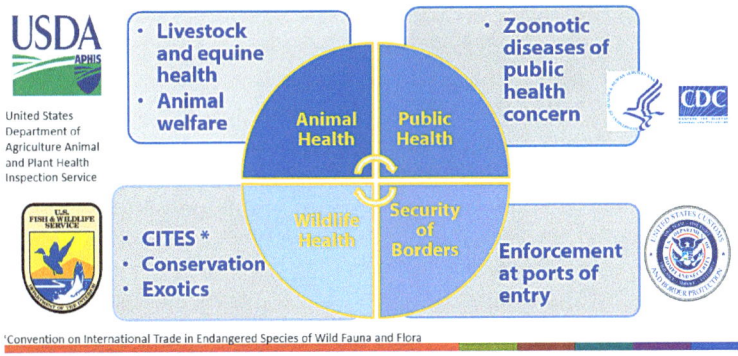

FIGURE 5-1 Federal governmental regulatory agencies for animal importation at ports of entry.
SOURCE: Brian Maskery, March 28, 2022.

---

[2] More information about the CDC Strategy for Global Response to COVID-19 can be found at https://www.cdc.gov/coronavirus/2019-ncov/global-COVID-19/global-response-strategy.html (accessed March 6, 2022).

[3] More information about the Runway to Recovery guidance can be found at https://www.transportation.gov/sites/dot.gov/files/2022-02/Runway_to_Recovery_1.1_DEC2020_Final-508.pdf (accessed March 6, 2022).

for complying with CDC guidance regarding COVID-19 and encourages data collection to support the CDC's contact tracing activities. The USCG coordinated efforts with CDC to facilitate the Conditional Sailing Order.[4] Gary Rasicot, acting assistant secretary of the CWMD at DHS, identified steps needed to enhance the partnership between DHS and the DGMQ: longer term solutions that do not rely on emergency funding; memorializing the CWMD Operational Support to the DGMQ; and augmenting feedback and adaptation (Rasicot, 2021).

DHS and the DGMQ partner in safeguarding national borders from the introduction and spread of infectious diseases. The United States has more than 320 ports of entry, 20 of which have CDC quarantine stations (Division of Global Migration and Quarantine, 2021). These quarantine stations are staffed with CDC medical and public health officers who coordinate medical treatment or cases and contact investigations with local public health and medical officials. DHS's CBP does initial screening of all travelers at all of the ports of entry including at preclearance ports located in a few other countries, for visible signs of illness. If CBP identifies a traveler that meets predetermined health risk criteria provided by the CDC, they refer those travelers to the CDC quarantine station staff. At the ports of entry where there are quarantine stations the DGMQ staff may sometimes perform this activity in person, and for all of the other points of entry (POEs) they support CBP remotely by telephone. While the 20 CDC quarantine stations cover all of the POEs, CBP officers serve as "eyes, ears, and hands for CDC and HHS." The DGMQ trains CBP officers to identify overt signs of quarantinable and other communicable diseases, which allows CBP officers to make an initial determination that a traveler may be ill. The CDC also provides job aids (RING cards) to support this function. The traveler is then referred to the CDC or a local public health official qualified to make a diagnosis. CBP staff do not diagnose illness; they only determine whether a traveler may be ill based on overtly identifiable signs or travel history (HHS and CDC, 2016; CRS, 2014). The DGMQ also collaborates with the CBP National Targeting Center to obtain passenger records to support contact tracing on flights where a traveler may have been ill (CBP, n.d.; DHS, 2020). The DGMQ also works with CBP to identify CDC-regulated animals, animal products, biologics, and human remains that pose a potential threat to human health and to ensure that CDC regulatory requirements are met (CBP, n.d.; DHS, 2020, 2022; Gursky and Batni, 2012; HHS and CDC, 2016; Seghetti, 2014).

---

[4] More information about the Conditional Sailing Order can be found at https://www.cdc.gov/quarantine/cruise/COVID19-cruiseships.html (accessed March 6, 2022).

Collaboration with the Transportation Security Administration

The DGMQ also coordinates with the TSA, which has responsibility for the security of private and commercial aviation. The TSA partners with the CDC/DGMQ in two important areas: by administering the Do Not Board list (CDC, 2022b) for certain infectious travelers who are noncompliant with local public health advice not to travel, and by issuing Security Directives and Emergency Amendments to impel commercial air carriers to implement measures consistent with CDC directives like a mask mandate. For individuals to be placed on the Do Not Board list, they have to be actively infectious, demonstrate they are noncompliant with public health isolation orders, and have an intent to board a commercial aircraft. If these criteria are met the DGMQ requests that the TSA put those individuals on a list that prevents them from obtaining a boarding pass.

The DGMQ also works with the TSA to implement certain public health measures in commercial aviation, such as the federal mandate requiring masking in airports and on all flights (CDC, 2022a; TSA, 2022). Additionally, the DGMQ works with USCIS to provide technical instructions and assistance for Civil Surgeons who perform required medical examinations for individuals seeking to change their immigration status within the United States (i.e., to become lawful permanent residents). Figure 5-2 illustrates the complementary missions of the DHS and the DGMQ.

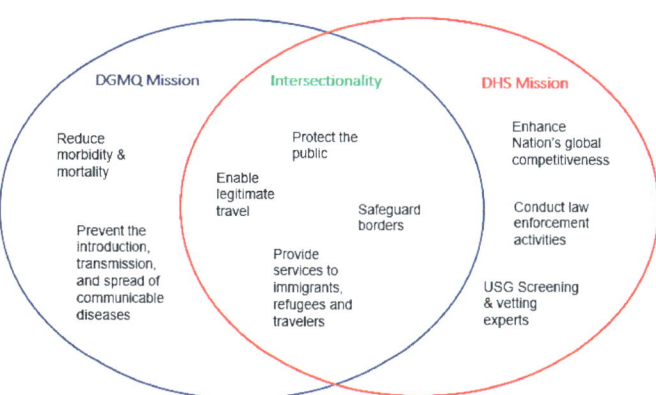

FIGURE 5-2 Complementary missions of the Department of Homeland Security and the Division of Global Migration and Quarantine.
NOTE: DGMQ = Division of Global Migration and Quarantine; DHS = Department of Homeland Security.
SOURCE: Rasicot, 2021.

Collaboration with the U.S. Department of Health and Human Services

The DGMQ works with the ORR to support refugee health programs for newly arrived refugees and it provides technical assistance regarding health programs for individuals staying at emergency intake sites while seeking asylum in the United States. The division also collaborates with the OGA on preparedness and response to pandemics and emerging threats and in addressing travel policies as part of the Global Health Security Initiative including the activities to strengthen U.S.–Mexico land border preparedness. The DGMQ also meets with Canadian counterparts monthly or more frequently (as has been the case during the COVID-19 pandemic) to engage in bilateral discussions, exchange information, or plan joint exercises (e.g., for an ill passenger on a train or bus). Additionally, it coordinated with the ACF to support individuals under federal quarantine or isolation orders after being repatriated from Wuhan, China, and during Operation Allied Welcome movement of persons from Afghanistan to the United States.

Collaboration with the U.S. Department of State

The DGMQ works with the DOS to support the required overseas immigrant and refugee medical examinations conducted by panel physicians. The DGMQ provides technical instructions and support to the panel physicians to conduct the exam. The DGMQ also works with the DOS on exemptions to COVID-related travel requirements (e.g., testing and vaccination requirements). The DGMQ also works with the DOS on preventive health programs (screening, vaccination, and presumptive treatment) for U.S.-bound refugees. The DGMQ provides information to the DOS to share with travelers via U.S. embassies regarding diseases of public health concern that may impact travelers and their pets.

Collaboration with Other Federal Partners

The DGMQ is responsible for regulating animals or animal products that pose a public health risk and restricting their entry to the United States (CDC, 2021c). In so doing, the DGMQ coordinates with other regulatory entities. Before the restriction of an animal or article is issued, the CDC must coordinate with other federal partners, including the USDA, the FDA (another partner within HHS), and the FWS (within DOI). The DGMQ works with the USDA and, specifically, APHIS to coordinate changes to animal and animal product importation regulations and to respond to importation events that result in denials of entry to the United States. This coordination aims to balance public health issues with private property rights, implications for the global economy and foreign relations, and public interests such as the availability of service animals for people with disabilities (HHS and CDC, 2016).

Collaboration with State, Local, Tribal, and Territorial Partners

Like its coordinated efforts with federal interagency partners, the DGMQ collaborations with various STLT partners are critical in preventing onward transmission of infectious diseases. Local and state jurisdictional health departments contribute to preventing and responding to infectious disease outbreaks in a range of invaluable ways, from surveillance activities to the deployment of immunizations to the delivery of screening, care, and treatment.

The HHS ASPR coordinates the overall public health response to a disease outbreak. If a public health event requires a federal response, the ASPR leads the National Response Framework Emergency Support Function (ESF) #8 (Public Health and Medical Services) (FEMA, 2008) on behalf of the HHS secretary. The ASPR spearheaded the medical countermeasure program through personnel deployment to support medical and quarantine facilities and provided needed equipment for surge demands in 2020 to protect the American population from COVID-19 spread (HHS, 2021). Through regular ESF8 conference calls and messages, ESF8 provides assistance to STLT partners. The National Association of County and City Health Officials (NACCHO) works to strengthen the capacities of local health departments to prevent and control the transmission of infectious diseases.[5] The Association of State and Territorial Health Officials (ASTHO) supports state and territorial public health agencies in outbreak response and prevention through the provision of immunization services and infectious disease prevention programs; its programmatic and policy work has a strong focus on improving health equity in the realm of infectious disease prevention and control.[6] The Council of State and Territorial Epidemiologists (CSTE) is also a key partner, particularly in the areas of developing public health policy and strengthening epidemiological capacity.[7] The Association of Public Health Laboratories (APHL) is also another important partner in building laboratory systems for detecting

---

[5] More information about NACCHO's work in infectious disease prevention and control is available from https://www.naccho.org/programs/community-health/infectious-disease (accessed March 8, 2022).

[6] More information about ASTHO's work in infectious disease prevention and control is available from https://www.astho.org/topic/infectious-disease (accessed March 8, 2022).

[7] More information about CSTE is available from https://www.cste.org/page/about-cste (accessed March 8, 2022).

public health threats across the nation and globally.[8] Although coordination and collaboration occur between federal and STLT partners, the CDC does not have legal authority over these entities for many of the needed public health responses.

Collaboration with International Partners

In working to mitigate the public health risks associated with global travel, the DGMQ collaborates with international partners. Much of this collaboration takes place in the division's Immigrant, Refugee, and Migrant Health (IRMH) branch, which strives to strengthen health systems at country borders and improve the health of immigrants, migrants, and refugees bound for the United States (CDC, 2021b). The IRMH branch's international partners include the World Health Organization (WHO); the United Nations Refugee Agency; the International Organization for Migration; and country governments, customs, immigration, and security agencies. International partners support the IRMH branch in conducting mandatory overseas medical examinations of immigrants and refugees, transmitting examination records to U.S. partner agencies and organizations, and facilitating continuity of care for these mobile populations. Additionally, the IRMH branch collaborates with international partners in border areas to develop technical capacities, including the development of tools to improve the collection and use of data to monitor population movement and disease spread. The United States–Mexico Unit (U.S. M.U.) of the DGMQ partners with Mexico's ministry of health to address multiple binational health issues related to the border region and maintains a field office in Mexico (CDC, 2019, 2021d).

International collaboration is highlighted in the CDC's National Center for Emerging and Zoonotic Infectious Diseases (NCEZID) 2018–2023 strategic plan, which includes the strategy to "improve international collaboration and capacities for emerging infectious disease prevention, surveillance, control and research" (NCEZID, 2018, pg. 11). Given its focus on international mobility, the DGMQ stands to play an important role in achieving this goal. Although international collaboration is essential in responding to global health risks, it is not easily achieved and involves tradeoffs during a crisis (Bump et al., 2021; Fry et al., 2020). The COVID-19 pandemic response demonstrated challenges to international collaboration that include (1) patterns of self-interested nationalism, particularly with regard to vaccine and medication access; (2) politicization of the pandemic response; (3) varying levels of collaboration between countries and WHO and other

---

[8] More information about APHL is available from https://www.aphl.org/aboutAPHL/Pages/default.aspx (accessed March 8, 2022).

multilateral agencies; (4) mistrust regarding data sharing; (5) institutional fragmentation; and (6) budgetary manipulation of WHO by some nations (Bump et al., 2021). Additionally, the time-sensitive nature of COVID-19 policy and research led to a prioritization of efficiency over collaboration (Fry et al., 2020).

The International Health Regulations (IHR) of 2005 are a mechanism for enhancing global collaboration for improved public health. The IHR are a legally binding framework of rights and obligations pertaining to public health events that have the potential to cross borders. These regulations outline the criteria of a "public health emergency of international concern" and include the requirements that countries establish and maintain surveillance and response capacities, report public health events, and comply with WHO communications expectations (WHO, n.d.).[9] Although the IHR have been adopted by 196 countries, their implementation requires substantial modifications in order to realize their potential (Gostin and Katz, 2016). The NCEZID 2018–2023 strategic plan underscored the importance of advancing the adoption of IHR and other global health policies in strengthening the global capacity to prevent, detect, and respond to international outbreaks of public health concern (NCEZID, 2018). The Committee received presentations indicating that many countries did not act in ways consistent with their IHR requirements, a further indication of the need for the IHR to be updated (Hoffman and Poirier, 2022). The U.S. government designated CDC quarantine stations as the competent authority to support the implementation of the IHR at U.S. POEs (CDC, 2021a). The quarantine stations are charged with preventing unwarranted restrictions on traffic and trade—thereby avoiding unnecessary disruptions—as they fulfill the responsibility of IHR implementation.

A special case of collaboration with international partners is the required interaction of the quarantine stations with agents across U.S. international land borders. This includes Mexican and Canadian public health agencies, ministries of health, and migration and travel-related authorities in those countries. Interactions occur regularly at the local level, but also include exchanges of information and other activities in agreement with the federal/national levels of those agencies and authorities. These public health and migration partnerships across the U.S.–Mexico and U.S.–Canada land borders allow the DGMQ to identify and respond to potential threats to public health. It also enables the DGMQ to locate people with confirmed cases of infectious diseases who need to be followed up once they enter U.S. territory.

---

[9] More information about the International Health Regulations is available from https://www.who.int/health-topics/international-health-regulations#tab=tab_1 (accessed March 9, 2022).

In the case of the Mexico–U.S. border, multiple cross-border coordination efforts are already in place, including initiatives such as the Binational Infectious Disease Surveillance (BIDS), the U.S.–Mexico Health Commission, and other ad hoc or sporadic activities such as capacity building, conferences, and public health investigation activities. The strength of collaboration between the CDC and its international partners in the region is thus based on a long-established relationship of the public health community on both sides of the border area. Still, according to public health experts who took part in a recent seminar on the impact of the COVID-19 pandemic on the border region, some challenges remain: (1) ensuring the sustainability of collaborations by ensuring that coordination mechanisms in both sides of the border have an adequate budget to continue operating; (2) moving forward toward the establishment of common protocols for surveillance and other public health actions at the border crossings and in the border regions; and (3) ensuring that the federal levels of each country understand and respond to the unique needs of border areas (Bojorquez-Chapela, in press; Fernández De Castro et al., in press).

Coordination with Airline and Maritime Industries

The DGMQ's role in preventing the introduction and transmission of infectious diseases into the United States involves coordination with airline and maritime industries. The Division's Quarantine Travel Epidemiology Team works with staff at the quarantine stations to respond to reports of illness or exposure to disease related to air or maritime travel when contact investigations are indicated. Its aviation activity works with STLT health departments, as well as with international partners, to facilitate aircraft contact investigations (Brown et al., 2021). Its Maritime Activity works with quarantine stations staff and maritime industry partners to respond to illnesses and outbreaks on ships as well as facilitate contact investigations among ship travelers. The majority of these illnesses—80 percent—take place on cruise ships, with the remaining 20 percent reported from cargo ships. The team facilitates maritime contact investigations among ship crew and passengers.[10] The DGMQ participated during the COVID-19 pandemic in industry calls coordinated by the FAA for airlines or by the DOT for surface transport to help industries remain informed about COVID-19 public health guidance and requirements and to provide a forum for engaging these industries.

Currently, the CDC collects information about airline passengers from CBP through the Advance Passenger Information System (APIS) and Passenger Name Records (PNR). Additionally, the airline industry is required

---

[10] This text was changed after release of the report to the study sponsor to clarify the role of DGMQ in maritime contact investigations.

to provide HHS and the CDC with any requested passenger data, according to the 2017 "Final Rule for Control of Communicable Diseases: Interstate and Foreign."[11] The final rule does not impose any new burdens on the airline industry. Instead, it codifies the current practice of HHS/CDC receiving a passenger manifest, if needed, and being provided with any data in an airline's possession.

The COVID-19 pandemic response required increased screening measures. In January 2020 the CDC instituted an enhanced screening program to reduce the importation of COVID-19 into the United States and slow its spread (Dollard et al., 2020). With support from DHS, the CDC screened passengers arriving from countries with widespread transmission of SARS-CoV-2 or with symptoms of the virus. The CDC and the FAA issued joint occupational health and safety guidance for airline crew members.[12] This guidance delegated post-arrival management of crew members to airline occupational health programs.

The COVID-19 pandemic posed multiple challenges to the airline and maritime industries. A study that examined international governance, communication, and response found that the travel health system did not provide early and appropriate risk warnings and alerts concerning cruise ship travel during the COVID-19 pandemic, and that this led to increasing numbers of infections on cruise ships (Zhou et al., 2020). The study concluded that multilateral coordination, cooperation, and collaboration mechanisms are needed between governments, organizations, and industry to improve travel health. The DGMQ has an important role to play in the development of a better international approach to maritime and aviation systems infectious disease control.

Collaboration with Academic Partners

Lessons from past pandemic response efforts provide key insights for evaluating the effectiveness of measures and outcomes. Various quarantine and isolation measures were implemented during the 1918 influenza pandemic, which present an opportunity for understanding and forecasting the impact of similar measures in the current and future pandemics. Conduct-

---

[11] The 2017 Final Rule is codified at 42 CFR Part 70 (interstate spread) and Part 71 (spread from foreign countries into the United States). More information is available from https://www.govinfo.gov/content/pkg/FR-2017-01-19/pdf/2017-00615.pdf (p. 6919) (accessed March 9, 2022).

[12] More information about FAA and CDC guidance can be found at https://www.faa.gov/other_visit/aviation_industry/airline_operators/airline_safety/safo/all_safos/media/2020/SAFO20009.pdf and at https://www.cdc.gov/quarantine/air/managing-sick-travelers/ncov-airlines.html (accessed March 8, 2021).

ing studies on these past events will be critical to better understand the science behind the decisions including the economic cost of pandemic-related measures. Collaborating with academic institutions for research or establishing "Centers of Excellence" can play an important role in generating scientific evidence that will help inform political decisions around disease control activities for migration and quarantine activities.

BEST PRACTICES FOR IMPROVING COORDINATION AND COLLABORATION

Coordination between Federal and STLT Systems

Developing and implementing best practices for improving coordination between federal and STLT systems can help to bolster infectious disease response efforts. For instance, through collaboration with federal and STLT stakeholders, the CSTE has identified multiple opportunities to strengthen communication and coordination between the DGMQ, the Quarantine and Border Health Services Branch (QBHSB), and jurisdictional health departments. A 2019 CSTE evaluation identified strategies to improve the processes through which STLT epidemiologists report ill travelers with diseases of public health concern to the QBHSB (CSTE, 2019). The report recommends that the DGMQ (1) develop standardized protocols and algorithms for jurisdictional reporting to quarantine stations, (2) provide clarity and justification for all data requested for reporting cases, (3) convene annual meetings between jurisdictions and quarantine stations, (4) develop training and reference materials regarding jurisdictional reporting to the DGMQ/QBHSB, and (5) explore further opportunities to strengthen communication with STLT health departments. Recommendations specific to jurisdictional health departments include (1) onboarding and training new key staff on reporting cases to the QBHSB, (2) verifying that jurisdictions have accurate contact information for their respective quarantine stations, and (3) ensuring that the CDC's Emergency Operations Center is accessible to all staff for reporting outside of normal operational hours. As noted in Chapter 3, there is also substantial variation in jurisdictional capacity to offer resources for large scale isolation and quarantine measures that needs to be taken into consideration (Allen, 2022).

A subsequent CSTE study conducted in 2021 evaluated jurisdictional and federal public health responses to past and current outbreaks (e.g., Ebola, measles, SARS-CoV-2) to identify best practices and areas for improvement (CSTE, 2021). This evaluation found that standardizing processes, clarifying communications, and building relationships across the federal and STLT levels are foundational to improving public health responses to outbreaks; an overview of the report's key recommendations is provided in Table 5-1.

TABLE 5-1 Recommendations from Council of State and Territorial Epidemiologists to CDC on Outbreak Response

Domain	Recommendation	Entity
Outbreak Response	Reduce multiple instances of communication by requesting all missing data elements for infectious traveler notifications at one time.	CDC
	Build a strong working relationship with jurisdictions and quarantine stations through regular communication and check-in meetings.	CDC
	Ensure that information sent to jurisdictions for follow-up is sent within the actionable period.	CDC
	Ensure call center surge staff are cross trained on other outbreaks.	CDC
	Develop shorter, on-demand webinar training for various outbreak response topics including awareness of HD local realities.	CDC
	Develop clear protocols, requirements, and data collection tools for jurisdictional health departments in the Do Not Board process.	CDC
	Address delays partners face when calling EOC call center.	CDC
CSTE Notification Protocol	Add link to CSTE Notification Protocol and Optional Form to DGMQ website.	CDC
Information Sharing	Create a secure, bidirectional portal for submitting/sharing information to improve timeliness and efficiency, especially for data that requires public health action.	CDC
	Develop a standardized data dictionary to allow jurisdictions to export data directly from their case management systems instead of manually completing the form for large volumes.	CDC
	Ensure there is ability to submit infectious traveler notifications in "batch" notifications for large volumes.	CDC
	Identify minimum data requirements and review current forms health departments use to submit multiple cases.	CDC

SOURCE: CSTE, 2021. https://cdn.ymaws.com/www.cste.org/resource/resmgr/crosscuttingi/Evaluation_of_Jurisdictional.pdf (accessed March 20, 2022).

Communication with Jurisdictions

To ensure clear and effective communication during emerging or ongoing outbreaks, the DGMQ needs to engage with jurisdiction-level stakeholders on a regular basis. An example of a successful partnership in outbreak response spanning the international, federal, and jurisdictional levels is Operation Allies Welcome (OAW), which was executed during the COVID-19 pandemic (Brown et al., 2021). On August 29, 2021, President Biden directed DHS to lead a humanitarian mission across multiple federal agencies to safely resettle vulnerable Afghans and U.S. citizens/legal permanent residents in the United States (DHS, 2021). DHS established a Unified Coordination Group (UCG) to coordinate the implementation of a large suite of services, including initial processing, COVID-19 testing, isolation of COVID-positive individuals, vaccinations, and additional medical services. The CDC staff supported OAW at three points of entry: Philadelphia (PHL), Washington Dulles (IAD), and Chicago O'Hare (ORD). During OAW Phase 1 (August 17–September 10, 2021), an estimated 63,430 travelers were supported in PHL and IAD. The operation paused after the identification and confinement of a measles outbreak in September, then resumed on October 4 to support 59 unaccompanied minors. During Phase 2, which began on October 5 and remains ongoing, an estimated 14,150 travelers had been supported as of October 31, 2021 (Brown et al., 2021).

The success of OAW has depended on communication and coordination across a range of international, federal, and STLT partners. State and local health departments assisted with mission coordination early on, as well as supporting the processes of testing, isolation, and quarantine. For the first 1–2 weeks, before DHS took over, the Office of Emergency Affairs of the Commonwealth of Virginia provided mission coordination.[13] During Phase 1, all Afghan evacuees (aged > 2 years) who arrived at IAD or PHL received onsite SARS-CoV-2 testing performed by the Virginia Department of Health (VDH) and Philadelphia Department of Public Health (PDPH), respectively, with support from a contracting agency. During Phase 2, only symptomatic travelers were tested. The VDH and PDPH also facilitated isolation and quarantine measures, as well as providing follow-up for all positive cases (limited to U.S. citizens/legal permanent residents) and their families. To enhance communication, evacuees were provided with educational materials in their native languages of Dari and Pashto (Brown et al., 2021).

ELEMENTS OF EFFECTIVE COORDINATION AND COLLABORATION

Robust coordination and collaboration at the national, regional, and local levels provide the foundation for timely and effective public health response to an emerging or ongoing outbreak of infectious disease. At the outset of the COVID-19 pandemic, Taiwan implemented a strategy

---

[13] This text was modified after release of the report to the study sponsor to correctly identify the partner.

of "collaborative governance" that underpinned the nation's successful collective response effort, which resulted in relatively low rates of SARS-CoV-2 infection and COVID-19 mortality compared to neighboring countries (Huang, 2020). Key elements of the collaborative governance model include cooperation between central and local governments, coordination with nongovernmental organizations and associations, and collaboration across sectors.

A 2021 study of the Dallas–Fort Worth public health and emergency management response to the 2014 Ebola outbreak identified essential components of effective coordination at the regional level (Soujaa et al., 2021). These components include an identifiable lead agency that coordinates policy, manages a network of organizations, and is authorized by a higher-level entity to use leverage and incentives to shape local action. A formal statement from local authorities regarding efforts made to address the health emergency was found to enhance efficacy of coordination. An environment conducive to informal communications—which can exist concurrently with formal structures—was found to generate flexibility and adaptation for effective coordination. The study also identified the following communication activities as essential for coordination: informing professionals of important developments and operations relevant to the crisis response, connecting professionals with one another, and involving the appropriate responders in decision-making processes.

To improve effectiveness of the federal policies before they are handed down, it is essential to actively engage with STLT public health partners to seek and incorporate their input when developing those policies. For example, in conjunction with CDC and DGMQ experts, the CSTE developed and updated a *Notification Protocol and Data Collection Guidance* to support health departments in notifying infectious persons with recent travel to the CDC's quarantine stations.[14] This process of seeking input from stakeholders at all levels should be continual throughout the cycle of response to an outbreak, beginning in the preparation phase before an outbreak occurs, then extending throughout the acute response and recovery stages. Existing mechanisms can be leveraged to facilitate this engagement. Predecisional input from the NACCHO, ASTHO, CSTE, and APHL before public health guidance policies, protocols, and documents would help to ensure that the final materials are realistic, practical, and effective.

In order to improve international collaboration to fulfill the DGMQ's goals, some elements proven to be relevant for successful partnerships should be considered. A commitment to common, measurable goals

---

[14] The most recent version of the *Notification Protocol and Data Collection Guidance* is available from https://cdn.ymaws.com/www.cste.org/resource/resmgr/crosscuttingi/CSTE_Notification_Protocol_a.pdf (accessed March 8, 2022).

serves as the foundation for the partnership (Bertolo et al., 2018). The scope, objectives, and strategies of effective partnerships are clearly defined and tailored to current need (Druce and Harmer, 2004). Components of scope in the public health context include disease, geography, population, and activities. Partnerships should have clear governance—with roles of all partners defined—and should feature inclusivity and representation of all stakeholders. Partnership processes should be respectful of cultural differences and flexible to allow for responsiveness to political, economic, and other changes in the environment. Trust and transparency foster consensus generation within partnerships. Efficient and effective partnerships align methodologies, share data, and utilize evidence-based approaches (Bertolo et al., 2018). A data-driven systems approach to global collaboration can ensure scientific integrity and improve efficiency (Ros et al., 2021).

Communication of Information to Travelers at Ports of Entry

Communication with travelers at U.S. POEs is a critical component of controlling the spread of infectious disease, both across and within national borders. The committee has identified a set of best practices to improve clarity and effectiveness in communicating information about ongoing or emerging infectious disease threats to incoming travelers at POEs. Key components of these best practices include predecisional collaboration and regular communication among international, federal, and STLT partners to ensure smooth operations on the ground at the jurisdictional level.

Predecisional Collaboration

Predecisional collaboration is foundational to infectious disease prevention and control efforts. As with policy and protocol development, perspectives and input from the full range of stakeholders and partners should be obtained through a robust and collaborative engagement process before any decisions or policies are finalized. This is especially critical for STLT partner agencies, as the implementation of prevention and control measures mostly occur at the state and local levels. Predecisional input can be coordinated through the major public health partner organizations, including the ASTHO, NACCHO, CSTE, and APHL. During other infectious disease outbreaks prior to the COVID-19 pandemic, this engagement process was conducted through existing mechanisms during the initial stages of the outbreaks. However, as those outbreaks progressed, this engagement process was either absent or inconsistently executed.

CONCLUSIONS AND RECOMMENDATIONS

Conclusions

Conclusion 5-1: To ensure that policies developed at the federal level are effective, it is important to incorporate input from state, tribal, local (county and city), and territorial health agencies and private sector entities.

Conclusion 5-2: Coordination and harmonization between localities will be critical in managing emergencies and outbreaks.

Conclusion 5-3: More effective and sustained engagement with regulated industries, such as maritime and aviation industries, is clearly needed.

Conclusion 5-4: International collaboration is an important component of the DGMQ's activities. The main framework for international collaboration regarding disease control and prevention are the International Health Regulations (IHR). However, the COVID-19 pandemic has demonstrated the need for the IHR to evolve in order to respond to future public health emergencies on a global scale. Since the DGMQ is the division within the CDC responsible for implementing the IHR, the DGMQ needs to play a major role in the ongoing revision of the IHR.

Conclusion 5-5: Interactions with international partners at the borders comprise another major element of the DGMQ's international collaboration. Successful collaboration requires the development of trust between partners, which is most effectively achieved through ongoing contact and opportunities to exchange views and define common goals. Different collaboration initiatives have already been developed in this region. However, increasing the continuity of those initiatives is important in fostering the development of trust over time, in making information exchange more regular and standardized, and in establishing common protocols. The DGMQ could play a major role in better understanding the unique needs of border regions at the federal level and the potential impact of these needs on the ability to detect and contain the spread of disease.

Conclusion 5-6: Promoting university/academic partnerships for collaborative research and evaluation, including establishing "Centers of Excellence in Global Migration and Quarantine," would enhance the knowledge base for disease control activities for migration and quarantine activities.

Conclusion 5-7: The DGMQ would benefit from the establishment of a formal federal advisory committee to provide external input on quarantine and border health issues on a regular and ongoing basis. Committee membership could include state and local officials, international partners, representatives from regulated industries, academic and private sector experts, professional societies, nongovernmental organizations and have ex-officio membership from other federal agencies.

Recommendations

Recommendation 5-1: The Division of Global Migration and Quarantine (DGMQ) should strengthen partnerships through defined and planned activities that enhance working relationships and continue to build trust.

To do so, the DGMQ should implement these specific measures:
A. Improve collaboration with international partners through regularly scheduled forums:
   1. Actively engage in the International Health Regulations (IHR) revision process.
   2. Ensure the continuity of binational collaborations in border areas to facilitate the development of trust between partners.
   3. Participate with other agencies and partners in the development and implementation of a harmonized approach to border measures with Mexico and Canada that features common protocols for disease surveillance and response in border areas.
B. Improve coordination between federal, state, tribal, local (county and city) and territorial (STLT) health agencies and strengthen international collaboration and engagement of quarantine officers.
   1. Develop a Federal Interagency Workgroup with input from STLT partners.
   2. Strengthen isolation and quarantine preparedness planning.
      a. Define federal and STLT roles and responsibilities.
      b. Understand and plan for variation in how STLT entities implement public health legal authorities.
      c. Implement a federal and STLT tabletop exercise program to bring together relevant quarantine stakeholders to practice coordination periodically, especially in regions containing quarantine stations.

3. Ensure pre-decisional input and engagement from STLT health agencies. It is critically important that DGMQ guidance and documents are informed by ground-level local (county and city) health agencies.
    a. Work to align DGMQ interventions with local public health activities to avoid overburdening the local public health system.
C. Improve coordination with aviation and maritime industries for border/traveler health issues and mandates:
    1. Build on coordination mechanisms established during the COVID-19 pandemic between aviation and maritime industries with STLT health agencies and the DGMQ. Examples of mechanisms for coordination include an Interagency Federal Workgroup, Memoranda of Agreement (MOA), Standard Operating Procedures (SOPs), emergency planning, drills, and exercises.
    2. Improve DGMQ engagement with regulated industries (e.g., cruise ship lines).
        a. Establish clear and consistent structure for communication.
        b. Develop clear objectives (e.g., safety and relative risk).
        c. Share and evaluate best practices at domestic and international ports.

Recommendation 5-2: The Division of Global Migration and Quarantine (DGMQ) should modernize health communication efforts with and for travelers to improve public understanding of disease control efforts as well as compliance.
   A. Develop standardized communication for travelers, families of travelers, and the general public (e.g., what to expect when traveling to the United States) to ensure that travelers understand and change behaviors to follow disease control and prevention measures.
   B. Establish mechanisms to utilize airlines, airport authorities, and travel agencies to communicate messages and better inform travelers during a pandemic, emerging pandemic, or outbreak.
   C. Collaborate with the aviation industry to provide pre-departure education and information sharing prior to flight boarding and during ticket purchase.
   D. Incorporate international best practices for communicating with passengers and sharing information regarding quarantine and testing requirements.

E. Incorporate avenues for the DGMQ to share informative materials with travelers in addition to the DGMQ website.
   1. Consider the use of electronic means of communication—such as flexible text messaging tools—to reach travelers with follow-up instructions and information.
F. In order to avoid health inequities, make these communications accessible for all travelers, regardless of language, access to technologies (e.g., smartphones), disabilities, and so on.

REFERENCES

Allen, M. 2022. *Enhancing the Federal Quarantine Station network—A state perspective: ASTHO*. Presentation to the National Academies of Sciences, Engineering, and Medicine Committee on Analysis to Enhance the Effectiveness of the Federal Quarantine Station Network.

Bertolo, R. F., E. Hentges, M.-J. Makarchuk, A. K. A. Wiggins, H. Steele, J. Levin, A. Grantham, L. Gramlich, and D. W. L. Ma. 2018. Key attributes of global partnerships in food and nutrition to align research agendas and improve public health. *Applied Physiology, Nutrition, and Metabolism* 43(7):755-758. https://doi.org/10.1139/apnm-2017-0715.

Bojorquez-Chapela, I. In press. Health systems in the San Diego-Tijuana region during the COVID-19 pandemic.

Brown, C., F. Alvarado-Ramy, and A. Klevos. 2021. *To screen or not to screen? There's more to border health than interventions at our borders: CDC*. Presentation to the National Academies of Sciences, Engineering, and Medicine Committee on Analysis to Enhance the Effectiveness of the Federal Quarantine Station Network.

Bump, J. B., P. Friberg, and D. R. Harper. 2021. International collaboration and COVID-19: What are we doing and where are we going? *BMJ* 372:n180. https://doi.org/10.1136/bmj.n180.

CBP (U.S. Customs and Border Protection). n.d. *Working together*. https://www.cbp.gov/frontline/cbp-national-targeting-center (accessed March 8, 2022).

CDC (Centers for Disease Control and Prevention). 2019. *United States–Mexico public health binational partnerships*. https://www.cdc.gov/usmexicohealth/binational-partnerships.html (accessed March 7, 2022).

CDC. 2021a. *Division of Global Migration and Quarantine Laws and Regulations*. Division of Global Migration and Quarantine (DGMQ). https://www.cdc.gov/ncezid/dgmq/laws-and-regulations.html (accessed May 19, 2022).

CDC. 2021b. *Immigrant, Refugee, and Migrant Health Branch*. Division of Global Migration and Quarantine (DGMQ). https://www.cdc.gov/ncezid/dgmq/focus-areas/irmh.html (accessed February 16, 2022).

CDC. 2021c. *Quarantine and Border Health Services*. Division of Global Migration and Quarantine (DGMQ). https://www.cdc.gov/ncezid/dgmq/focus-areas/quarantine.html (accessed February 28, 2022).

CDC. 2021d. *United States–Mexico health*. Division of Global Migration and Quarantine (DGMQ). https://www.cdc.gov/ncezid/dgmq/focus-areas/usmh.html (accessed May 19, 2022).

CDC. 2022a. *Air travel toolkit for airline partners*. https://www.cdc.gov/coronavirus/2019-ncov/travelers/airline-toolkit.html (accessed March 12, 2022).

CDC. 2022b. *Travel restrictions to prevent the spread of disease.* https://www.cdc.gov/quarantine/travel-restrictions.html (accessed March 12, 2022).
CRS (Congressional Research Service). 2014. CRS report r43356: Border security: Immigration inspections at ports of entry. Congressional Research Service. https://sgp.fas.org/crs/homesec/R43356.pdf (accessed May 15, 2022).
CSTE (Council of State and Territorial Epidemiologists). 2019. *Evaluation of reports of ill travelers to Quarantine and Border Health Services Branch.* https://www.cste.org/members/group.aspx?id=87618 (accessed March 20, 2022).
CSTE. 2021. *Evaluation of jurisdictional & federal public health responses to past & current outbreaks & implementation of CSTE protocol for health department notification to CDC quarantine stations of infectious persons with recent travel.* Atlanta, Georgia: Council of State and Territorial Epidemiologists. https://cdn.ymaws.com/www.cste.org/resource/resmgr/crosscuttingi/Evaluation_of_Jurisdictional.pdf (accessed March 20, 2022).
DHS (Department of Homeland Security). 2020. *Privacy impact assessment for the CBP support of CDC for public health contact tracing.* https://www.dhs.gov/sites/default/files/publications/privacy-pia-cbp056-cdccontactracing-december2020.pdf (accessed March 15, 2022).
DHS. 2021. *Operation Allies Welcome.* https://www.dhs.gov/allieswelcome (accessed March 8, 2022).
DHS. 2022. *Congressional budget justification FY 2022: U.S. Customs and Border Protection.* Washington, DC: U.S. Department of Homeland Security. https://www.dhs.gov/publication/congressional-budget-justification-fy-2022 (accessed May 19, 2022).
Division of Global Migration and Quarantine. 2021. *Immigrant, Refugee, and Migrant Health Branch.* https://www.cdc.gov/ncezid/dgmq/focus-areas/irmh.html (accessed May 22, 2022).
Dollard, P., I. Griffin, A. Berro, N. J. Cohen, K. Singler, Y. Haber, C. de la Motte Hurst, A. Stolp, S. Atti, L. Hausman, C. E. Shockey, S. Roohi, C. M. Brown, L. D. Rotz, M. S. Cetron, CDC COVID-19 Port of Entry Team, and F. Alvarado-Ramy. 2020. Risk assessment and management of COVID-19 among travelers arriving at designated U.S. airports, January 17–September 13, 2020. *MMWR: Morbidity and Mortality Weekly Report* 69(45):1681-1685. http://dx.doi.org/10.15585/mmwr.mm6945a4.
Druce, N., and A. Harmer. 2004. *The determinants of effectiveness: Partnerships that deliver review of the GHP and "business" literature.* London, UK: DFID Health Resource Centre. https://www2.ohchr.org/english/issues/development/docs/WHO_6.pdf (accessed March 6, 2022).
FEMA (Federal Emergency Management Agency). 2008. *Emergency support function #8—public health and medical services annex.* Hyattsville, MD: FEMA. https://www.fema.gov/sites/default/files/2020-07/fema_ESF_8_Public-Health-Medical.pdf (accessed May 22, 2022).
Fernández De Castro, R., P. Ganster, and C. González Gutiérrez. In press. Calibaja: Emerging stronger after COVID-19.
Fry, C. V., X. Cai, Y. Zhang, and C. S. Wagner. 2020. Consolidation in a crisis: Patterns of international collaboration in early COVID-19 research. *PLOS ONE* 15(7):e0236307. https://doi.org/10.1371/journal.pone.0236307.
Gostin, L. O., and R. Katz. 2016. The International Health Regulations: The governing framework for global health security. *The Milbank Quarterly* 94(2):264-313. https://doi.org/10.1111/1468-0009.12186.
Gursky, E., and S. Batni. 2012. *Failures at the nexus of health and homeland security: The 2007 Andrew Speaker case, Case studies working group report.* Carlisle, PA: Strategic Studies Institute, U.S. Army War College.

HHS (U.S. Department of Health and Human Services). 2021. *ASPR takes action to protect the nation from COVID-19 and other public health threats*. https://www.phe.gov/about/review-2020/Pages/default.aspx (accessed May 22, 2022).

HHS and CDC. 2016. *Notice of proposed rulemaking, control of communicable diseases, CDC Docket No. CDC-2016-0068*. Washington, DC: *The Federal Register*.

Hoffman, S. J., and M. J. P. Poirier. 2022. *The law, epidemiology and politics of COVID-19 national border closures*. Global Strategy Lab. Presentation to the National Acadmies of Sciences, Engineering, and Medicine Committee on Analysis to Enhance the Effectiveness of the Federal Quarantine Station Network.

Huang, I. Y.-F. 2020. Fighting COVID 19 through government initiatives and collaborative governance: The Taiwan experience. *Public Administration Review* 80(4):665-670. https://doi.org/10.1111/puar.13239.

NCEZID (National Center for Emerging and Zoonotic Infectious Diseases). 2018. *National Center for Emerging and Zoonotic Infectious Diseases Strategic Plan: 2018–2023*. https://www.cdc.gov/ncezid/pdf/ncezid-strategic-plan-2018-2023-508.pdf (accessed March 4, 2022).

Rasicot, G. 2021. *DHS support to DGMQ: A collaborative approach*. Presentation to the National Acadmies of Sciences, Engineering, and Medicine Committee on Analysis to Enhance the Effectiveness of the Federal Quarantine Station Network.

Ros, F., R. Kush, C. Friedman, E. Gil Zorzo, P. Rivero Corte, J. C. Rubin, B. Sanchez, P. Stocco, and D. Van Houweling. 2021. Addressing the COVID 19 pandemic and future public health challenges through global collaboration and a data driven systems approach. *Learning Health Systems* 5(1):e10253. https://doi.org/10.1002/lrh2.10253.

Seghetti, L. 2014. *Border security: Immigration inspections at ports of entry*. Washington, DC: Congressional Research Service. https://sgp.fas.org/crs/homesec/R43356.pdf (accessed May 22, 2022).

Soujaa, I., J. A. Nukpezah, and A. D. Benavides. 2021. Coordination effectiveness during public health emergencies: An institutional collective action framework. *Administration & Society* 53(7):1014-1045. https://dx.doi.org/10.1177/0095399720985440.

TSA (Transportation Security Administration). 2022. *Statement regarding face mask use on public transportation*. https://www.tsa.gov/news/press/statements/2022/04/18/statement-regarding-face-mask-use-public-transportation#:~:text=Due%20to%20today's%20court%20ruling,public%20transportation%20and%20transportation%20hubs (accessed May 5, 2022).

WHO (World Health Organization). n.d. *International health regulations*. https://www.who.int/health-topics/international-health-regulations#tab=tab_1 (accessed March 7, 2022).

Zhou, S., L. Han, P. Liu, and Z.-J. Zheng. 2020. Global health governance for travel health: Lessons learned from the coronavirus disease 2019 (COVID-19) outbreaks in large cruise ships. *Global Health Journal* 4(4):133-138. https://doi.org/10.1016/j.glohj.2020.11.006.

6

Legal and Regulatory Authority

The Centers for Disease Control and Prevention (CDC) exercised broad regulatory authority throughout the COVID-19 pandemic, with many of its actions challenged in, or even blocked by, the courts. The committee believes that the CDC should be afforded ample legal authority to carry out its mission using evidence-based measures to reduce the interstate or international spread of infectious diseases. This would require legal reforms, including modernizing the Public Health Service Act of 1944 (PHSA),[1] which was enacted well before major societal changes—including globalization—that can amplify the threat of rapidly moving infectious diseases. In addition to statutory reform, the CDC may also have to update its regulations to better respond to emerging health threats and include use of digital technology for contact tracing and monitoring to enable their use while respecting rights to privacy and freedom of movement. This chapter discusses potential changes to laws and regulations that may be required to implement recommended measures on infrastructure, workforce, data systems, as well as important reforms to ensure the CDC has the powers required to safeguard the American public.

---

[1] Public Health Service Act of 1944, Public Law 78-410, 78th Cong., 2nd sess. (July 1, 1944), 42.

THE CDC'S LEGAL AND REGULATORY AUTHORITY DURING OUTBREAKS: OVERVIEW

The PHSA authorizes the secretary of the Department of Health and Human Services (HHS) to take regulatory action[2] to prevent the introduction and spread of infectious diseases; this authority has subsequently been delegated to the CDC.

The Agency's Division of Global Migration and Quarantine (DGMQ) is responsible for drafting regulations and undertakes operations related to this regulatory authority. These include the authority to test, medically examine, detain, and release persons entering the United States who are suspected of carrying communicable diseases, including passengers and crew members (CDC, 2021c). The DGMQ provides this operational support through its work at U.S. ports of entry, by administering interstate and foreign quarantine regulations, and developing requirements for the testing, medical examination, and treatment of immigrants and refugees (CDC, 2021b). Together, the PHSA and Immigration and Nationality Act of 1952[3] and the PHSA authorize the federal government to develop medical examination requirements for immigrants and refugees entering the United States (CDC, 2021b). The Immigrant, Refugee, and Migrant Health branch of the DGMQ establishes medical screening protocols for physicians and other health care professionals to use worldwide in conducting medical examinations before individuals arrive in the United States to visit, live, and/or work.

The CDC is authorized to issue a federal isolation or quarantine order if a quarantinable disease[4] is suspected or identified (CDC, 2021c). Additionally, the CDC has the authority to restrict the importation of animals, animal products, human remains, or any other items that may pose public health threats. The U.S. quarantine stations also have the authority to implement the International Health Regulations (IHR) of 2005 which the World Health Organization (WHO) adopted to support global health security. The IHR, revised in 2005 in the aftermath of the SARS outbreaks, have been adopted by 196 countries, including the United States. While safeguarding global health security, the IHR also seek to prevent unwarranted travel and trade restrictions that might unnecessarily disrupt traffic and trade (CDC, 2021b; Gostin, 2021)

---

[2] These federal regulations apply to all persons, vehicles, animals regulated by the CDC, articles, and human remains entering the United States from another country by land, air, or sea.

[3] *Immigration and Nationality Act of 1952*, Public Law 82-414, 82nd Cong., 2nd sess. (June 27, 1952).

[4] Diseases are established as quarantinable by way of executive order of the president. More information about quarantinable diseases can be found at https://www.cdc.gov/quarantine/aboutlawsregulationsquarantineisolation.html (accessed March 2, 2022).

The congressional authorization of the CDC's regulatory powers may be interpreted broadly or narrowly. A broad interpretation of the PHSA would allow the CDC to adopt most evidence-based prevention or response measures that are constitutionally permissible for a federal executive-branch agency. In recent rulings enjoining some of the CDC's COVID-19 orders related to the CDC's repeated issuance of eviction moratoriums, however, the Supreme Court and several lower federal courts have indicated that the CDC's statutory authority be interpreted far more narrowly. Some lower courts have also held that Congress is constitutionally prohibited from delegating authority to administrative agencies in broad, catch-all terms. The U.S. Supreme Court has intimated in existing opinions that it may endorse a similar constitutional approach in the near future (Gostin et al., 2022). If the CDC is to be able to exercise powers to protect the public's health, it will likely require congressional reforms of the PHSA.

Uncertainty about the scope and limits of CDC authority could hinder pandemic prevention and response. Congress should modernize the CDC's powers by specifying the conditions under which it may, inter alia, (1) regulate interstate and international travel, (2) require use of personal protective equipment (PPE), (3) mandate sanitation measures, (4) limit mass gatherings, (5) regulate gathering places, or (6) adopt protections to support compliance with public health guidance. In addition, the CDC should initiate rulemaking building on the 2017 revised rules to clarify the standards and procedures governing such orders. This chapter first describes the sources and uses of the CDC's powers and recent court rulings enjoining its orders. This is followed by a discussion of reforms recommended by the committee to ensure the CDC's powers are comprehensive, constitutional, effective, and flexible. The Committee also suggests reforms to safeguard constitutionally protected individual rights, such as rights to privacy, assembly, travel, and liberty.

RECENT COURT INTERPRETATIONS OF THE CDC'S AUTHORITY

Recent court rulings have contributed to uncertainty regarding the scope of the CDC's authority. The PHSA gives the CDC powers to prevent the international and interstate spread of communicable disease. In addition to authorizing certain containment measures in specific terms (e.g., detention of international travelers and decontamination of articles in interstate commerce), Congress authorized "other measures" officials deem "necessary."[5] Recent court rulings have interpreted this language narrowly, limiting the CDC to measures "similar to" those specifically listed,[6] which "directly relate to preventing the interstate spread of disease by identifying,

---

[5] Public Health Service Act of 1944.
[6] *Tiger Lily, LLC v. Dep't of Housing and Urban Dev.*, 5 F.4th 666, 671 (6th Cir. 2021).

isolating, and destroying the disease itself."[7] These rulings were preliminary, but appeals that could lead to final decisions on the merits may be dismissed on procedural grounds as moot. Thus, the scope of the CDC's authority—particularly when narrowly targeted containment efforts fail—is uncertain. At the same time, the Supreme Court has interpreted certain federal agency powers narrowly, such as its decision in January 2022 to block the Occupational Safety and Health Administration's (OSHA's) vaccinate-or-test mandate for large employers (Gostin et al., 2022).

Specific and Broadly Delineated Powers Granted by the Public Health Service Act

The PHSA grants the CDC a combination of specific and broadly delineated powers. Sections 361 and 362 of the PHSA[8] authorize federal health officials[9] "to prevent the introduction, transmission, or spread of communicable diseases" into the United States from foreign countries and across state and territorial borders within the United States. These provisions are in a part of the PHSA titled "Quarantine and Inspection." However, they authorize at least some additional measures.

Congress granted the CDC some powers in specific terms; others are more broadly delineated. The first sentence of Subsection 361(a) is framed broadly. It states that the CDC director is "authorized to make and enforce *such regulations as in his judgment are necessary* to prevent the introduction, transmission, or spread of communicable diseases from foreign countries into the States or possessions, or from one State or possession into any other State or possession." The second sentence of Subsection 361(a) provides a nonexhaustive list of specific measures that are authorized by the first sentence: "For purposes of carrying out and enforcing such regulations, the [CDC director] may provide for such inspection, fumigation, disinfection, sanitation, pest extermination, destruction of animals or articles found to be so infected or contaminated as to be sources of dangerous infection to human beings, *and other measures, as in his judgment may be necessary*." Subsections 361(b) through (d) refer specifically to the use of Subsection 361(a) powers to apprehend, detain, examine, and conditionally release individuals and impose particular conditions on these measures. Section

---

[7] *Ala. Ass'n of Realtors v. Dep't of Health and Human Svcs.* 141 S.Ct. 2485, 2488 (2021).

[8] Sections 361 and 362 of the PHSA are codified at 42 U.S.C. §§264 and 265. This chapter uses the section numbering from the original legislation because that is how federal officials and lawmakers typically refer to these provisions.

[9] In 1944, Congress granted the powers discussed in this paper to the Surgeon General. In 1966, these powers were transferred to the secretary of Health and Human Services (HHS), who in turn delegated them to the CDC director and FDA commissioner. The FDA uses this authority to regulate "Section 361 products."

362 provides specific authority to prohibit introduction of persons or property into the United States from foreign countries designated by the CDC director. Additional provisions scattered throughout Title III of the PHSA set forth penalties for violations (Section 368), provide for acceptance of enforcement assistance from state and local officials (Section 311), and direct customs and Coast Guard officers to provide enforcement assistance (Section 365). Subsection 361(e)—which was added to the PHSA in 2002—provides that federal measures adopted under Section 361 preempt state and local laws that conflict with federal requirements.

The CDC has promulgated regulations interpreting these provisions most recently in 2017. The 2017 "Final Rule for Control of Communicable Diseases: Interstate and Foreign" is codified at 42 CFR Part 70 (interstate spread) and Part 71 (spread from foreign countries into the United States). Table 6-1 provides an overview of the major powers granted to the CDC by the PHSA. As with statutory reform, regulatory actions can be laborious and political. It took the CDC several iterations and more than a decade to finalize its 2017 Final Rule.

TABLE 6-1 Powers Granted to the CDC by the Public Health Service Act of 1944

Authority	Statute
Power to make and enforce regulations necessary to prevent the introduction, transmission, or spread of communicable diseases into the United States from foreign countries and across state and territorial borders within the United States.	PHSA Section 361(a)
Power to apprehend, detain, and conditionally release individuals to prevent inter- or intrastate cross-border spread of communicable diseases designated as quarantinable[a] by executive order.	PHSA Section 361(b)
Power to inspect, disinfect, and destroy animals and articles infected or contaminated by any communicable disease deemed "dangerous" to humans.	PHSA Section 361(a)
Power to implement border controls required in the interest of the public health to avert serious danger of the introduction of a communicable disease into the United States.	PHSA Section 362
Power to implement other "necessary measures" to prevent the spread of communicable disease into the United States from foreign countries or across state and territorial borders.	PHSA Section 361(a)

[a] Current list of quarantinable diseases: cholera, diphtheria, infectious tuberculosis, plague, smallpox, yellow fever, viral hemorrhagic fevers, severe acute respiratory syndromes, influenza viruses with pandemic potential, and measles.

Power to Apprehend, Detain, and Conditionally Release Individuals

Under Section 361(b), the CDC's power to apprehend, detain, or conditionally release individuals is triggered by a finding that these actions are necessary to prevent the cross-border spread of a communicable disease that the president has designated as quarantinable in an executive order. Currently, the list of quarantinable diseases is limited to cholera, diphtheria, infectious tuberculosis, plague, smallpox, yellow fever, viral hemorrhagic fevers, severe acute respiratory syndromes, influenza viruses with pandemic potential, and measles.[10] If the CDC sought to apprehend, detain, or conditionally release individuals based on the risk of any other communicable disease, the president would first have to issue an executive order amending the list of quarantinable diseases. The PHSA amendments in 2002 streamlined the process for updating the list. Section 361(c) specifies that these powers may be used to detain individuals entering the United States from a foreign country. Section 361(d) specifies that these powers may be used to detain individuals posing a risk of interstate spread only if the individual is "reasonably believed to be infected with a communicable disease in a qualifying stage" and "moving or about to move from" one state to another or "a probable source of infection" to other individuals who will be moving from one state to another while infected.

Regulations codified at 42 CFR §70.5, 70.6, 70.10, 70.12 et seq., and 71.29 et seq. (adopted in 2017) include extensive provisions to ensure the CDC orders for apprehension, screening, medical examination, isolation, quarantine, and conditional release are consistent with constitutional principles of federalism, separation of powers, and protections for individual rights (Gostin and Hodge, 2017).

Power to Inspect, Disinfect, and Destroy Animals and Articles

Under Section 361(a), the CDC may order "inspection, fumigation, disinfection, sanitation, pest extermination, [and] destruction of animals or articles" infected or contaminated by any communicable disease deemed "dangerous" to humans. Under 42 CFR §71.32, the CDC has determined this authority should only be used to prevent international spread if the disease is quarantinable. 42 CFR §70.2, which governs use of these measures to prevent interstate spread, is not limited to quarantinable diseases. It does, however, require a determination that the measures taken by state, territorial, and local health authorities are "insufficient to prevent" the interstate spread of disease.

---

[10] Exec. Order No. 13295 (Apr. 4, 2003) as amended by Exec. Order No. 13375 (Apr. 1, 2005); Exec. Order No. 13674 (Jul. 31, 2014); and Exec. Order No. 14047 (Sept. 17, 2021). 70 FR 17299.

Power to Implement Border Controls

Section 362 states that the CDC's power to prohibit, in whole or in part, "introduction of persons and property" from foreign countries designated by the CDC director is triggered by a finding that "by reason of the existence of any communicable disease in a foreign country there is serious danger of the introduction of such disease" into the United States. Additionally, CDC officials must find that the danger of introduction into the United States is "so increased by the introduction of persons or property" from the designated country or that border controls are "required in the interest of the public health." Border controls are authorized for the period of time deemed "necessary" to avert serious danger of the introduction of a communicable disease into the United States.

A regulation promulgated by the CDC clarifies the agency's interpretation of the scope and limits of its authority under Section 362. 42 CFR §71.40 narrows Section 362 by limiting its application to quarantinable diseases. However, the regulation also defines key terms in the statute broadly to maximize the measures the CDC may undertake to control quarantinable diseases. The regulation specifies that the CDC director's authority to "prohibit introduction" of persons "into the U.S." covers situations where the communicable disease at issue is already present within the United States and includes authority to "physically expel" individuals from the United States.

Power to Implement Other "Necessary Measures" to Prevent Cross-Border Disease Spread

The legislative history of the PHSA indicates that Congress intentionally chose broad language to authorize "other measures, as in [the CDC director's] judgement may be necessary" to prevent the spread of communicable disease into the United States from foreign countries or across state and territorial borders.[11] Administrative officials and judges may read

---

[11] A recent report by the Congressional Research Service notes that legislators viewed Section 361's broadly framed first sentence as a continuation of an 1893 statute authorizing "regulations to prevent the spread into the country, or between the States, of contagious or infectious diseases," but only if state and local regulations were nonexistent or inadequate. Act of Apr. 29, 1878 §5, ch. 66. The drafters of Section 361 understood that it would be "confined to matters pertaining to the interstate movement of people or things over which the States have both constitutional and practical difficulties in achieving effective control." However, they also emphasized that "these provisions are written in broader terms in order to make it possible to cope with emergency situations which we cannot now foresee" (Hearing Before a Subcomm. on Interstate & Foreign Commerce on H.R. 3379: A Bill to Codify the Laws Relating to the Public Health Service, and for Other Purposes, 78th Cong. 64 [1944]). In a committee hearing, the Surgeon General argued that Section 361 "may be very important because of the

this power narrowly or broadly. If it is read broadly, this language "might encompass the authority to implement any evidenced-based public health measures that do not . . . exceed constitutional limits."[12] The text of the PHSA does not limit the "necessary measures" provision to quarantinable communicable diseases.

The CDC's regulations implementing Section 361(a) provide minimal guidance regarding how this catch-all authority may be used. Under 42 CFR §70.2, the CDC's power to prevent the interstate spread of disease is conditioned on a determination "that the measures taken by [state, territorial, and local health authorities] are insufficient to prevent" the interstate spread of disease. In addition, §70.2 adopts a "reasonably necessary" standard to clarify that the PHSA's use of "necessary" does not require that the measure in question must be the only available means to an end.

The CDC's Regulatory Powers and Federal Emergency Declarations

The CDC powers previously described are not "emergency powers" per se. The PHSA and other statutes authorize federal officials to issue several distinct types of emergency and disaster declarations or determinations. Most relevant for the current purposes, Section 319(a) of the PHSA authorizes the HHS secretary to determine that "a) a disease or disorder presents a public health emergency (PHE); or b) that a public health emergency, including significant outbreaks of infectious disease or bioterrorist attacks, otherwise exists." A federal PHE determination allows the HHS secretary greater flexibility to suspend, waive, or modify certain regulatory requirements that might otherwise impede the health care system's emergency response, to make grants, to enter into contracts, and to access emergency and reserve funds. A PHE determination does not formally expand the CDC's statutory authorization in any way, but courts are likely to afford the CDC more deference in a declared health emergency. This differs from how state statutes typically authorize public health agencies to exercise a combination of general regulatory powers—which do not depend on a pending declaration—and emergency powers, which equip executive-branch officials with expanded delegations of authority while an emergency or disaster or PHE declaration is in effect. Although the HHS secretary's determination does not formally expand the CDC's regulatory

---

possibility that strange diseases may be introduced in the country and become a threat," and "[f]lexibility in dealing with such contingencies would be very helpful" (Hearing before a Subcomm. on Educ. and Labor, 78th Cong. 6 [1944]; Congressional Research Service, Scope of CDC Authority Under Section 361 of the Public Health Service Act [Apr. 13, 2021] at 9-10).

[12] Id. at 4.

powers, the CDC may choose to take the HHS secretary's PHE determination into account when determining whether a measure is "necessary" under Section 361 or 362.

CDC COVID-19 Orders Relying on Broad Interpretation of the Public Health Service Act

In the roughly 75 years since the CDC's founding and the PHSA's passage, the United States had not experienced a public health emergency of the scale and nature of the COVID-19 pandemic. During the response to the pandemic, the CDC has issued orders that have relied on a broad interpretation of the PHSA. In litigation defending its COVID-19 orders, the CDC has argued that judges should read Section 361 broadly to authorize restrictions and mandates for individuals, businesses, and airports, ports, and carriers—including face-mask requirements for public transit, vaccination requirements for cruise ships, testing requirements for air passengers entering the United States, and a moratorium on residential evictions. These measures were unprecedented for the CDC. The CDC had previously ordered targeted screening, isolation, and quarantine for containment and prevention purposes, but had rarely, if ever, ordered mitigation measures that apply to the general public in the absence of individualized risk assessment. An overview of orders issued by the CDC and operationalized with support from DGMQ is provided in Table 6-2.

Screening and Orders for Collection of Contact Information

Prior to and during the COVID-19 pandemic, Customs and Border Protection (CBP) performs most of the screening utilizing CDC protocols. However, the CDC has instituted screening programs for travelers entering the United States in circumstances of increased need for intervention. The CDC will screen with assistance from Customs and Border Protection[13] and has also issued orders requiring airlines to collect contact information for passengers arriving in the United States from specified foreign countries (Bajema et al., 2020; Brown et al., 2014). On October 25, 2021, the CDC issued an expanded order to collect contact information from all airline passengers en-

---

[13] See, e.g., Clive M. Brown et al., Airport Exit and Entry Screening for Ebola—August–November 10, 2014, 63 *Morbidity & Mortality Weekly Rpt.* 1163 (2014). Out of 256 individuals across 34 jurisdictions for whom CDC staff recommended SARS-CoV-2 testing in January 2020—at a time when testing was available in the United States solely through the CDC—six were identified through airport screening. The CDC has not specified whether any of the six identified through airport screening were among the 11 who tested positive in the United States in January 2020. See Kristina L. Bajema, et al.

TABLE 6-2 Orders issued by the DGMQ since COVID-19[a]

Order	Issue Date	Expiry Date
No Sail/Conditional-Sail Order	• No Sail: March 15, 2020 • Cond. Sail: October 30, 2020	January 15, 2022
Global Testing Order	• Original: January 2021 • Ukraine addition: April 2022 subject to extension as needed	
Safe Resumption of Global Travel	• November 2021 Amended in December 2021 to require all international travelers to be tested within 1 day prior to departure.	
Face Mask Order	February 2021	
Global Contact Tracing Order	February 7, 2020	Will cease to be in effect on the earlier of (1) the date that is two incubation periods after the last known case of 2019–nCoV, or (2) when the secretary determines there is no longer a need for this interim final rule
Suspension of Entry ("Title 42") Order	March 20, 2020	Will cease to be in effect on the earlier of (1) one year from the publication of this interim final rule, or (2) when the HHS secretary determines there is no longer a need for this interim final rule

[a] This table was modified after release of the report to the study sponsor to correct and provide specificity for the issue date and current status (as of June 6, 2022).

Current Status	Authority
• Optional but recommended participation in the CDC's Program for Cruise Ships	Under section 361 & 365 of the Public Health Service Act (42 U.S. Code §§264, 268)
• Ongoing • Temporary allowance of entry of Persons from Ukraine without a Pre-Departure test	Under Section 361 of the Public Health Service Act (42 U.S. Code §264) and 42 Code of Federal Regulations 71.20 and 71.31(b) and 71.32(b)
• Ongoing • CDC enforcement of the presidential proclamation requiring vaccination for noncitizen & nonimmigrants entering the United States	Sections 1182(f) and 1185(a)(1) of Title 8, and Section 301 of Title 3, United States Code, (the "Proclamation"), titled, "Advancing the Safe Resumption of Global Travel During the COVID–19 Pandemic."
• Ongoing but enforcement was suspended by a U.S. District Court judge • The CDC is reviewing the guidance and plans to make amendments to the current requirements.	Under Section 361 of the Public Health Service Act (42 U.S. Code §264) 42 Code of Federal Regulations 70.2, 71.31(b),
• Ongoing	Under Section 215 and 311 of the Public Health Service Act (42 U.S. Code R §71)
• The Order was terminated, but a U.S. District Court judge issued a preliminary injunction requiring continued enforcement.	Under Sections 362 of the Public Health Service Act (42 U.S. Code §265)

tering the United States from foreign countries.[14] This order replaced a series of prior orders that began in early 2020 applying to passengers arriving from specific countries. These activities rely on Section 361 and other authorities scattered throughout Title III of the PHSA, as implemented in 42 CFR §71.4.

Isolation and Quarantine Orders

The CDC has occasionally issued isolation and quarantine orders under Section 36, including an isolation order in 2007, for an individual believed to be infected with extensively drug-resistant tuberculosis (Parmet, 2007).[15] In late January 2020 the CDC issued quarantine orders—for the first time in more than 50 years—for 195 U.S. citizens whom the State Department repatriated from mainland China after they were believed to have been exposed to SARS-CoV-2 in Hubei province (CDC, 2020a,b). These orders rely on PHSA Sections 361(a) and (b).

Cruise Ship Operations

On March 14, 2020, as noted in Box 6-1, the CDC relied on Section 361(a) to issue an order suspending cruise ship operations from U.S. ports of call.[16] This order was extended until October 30, 2020, when the CDC replaced its "no-sail" order with a "conditional-sail" order[17] that set forth extensive sanitation, screening, and testing requirements for cruise ship operators before the CDC would permit them to resume sailing. Cruise operators could avoid the requirement to complete a "test sail" without paying passengers by ensuring at least 98 percent of crew and 90 percent of passengers were fully vaccinated (CDC, 2022b).

The CDC did not tether rescission of the March 2020 no-sail order to rescission of the HHS secretary's PHE declaration, which was first issued on January 31, 2020, and remains in effect as of this writing. In October 2020, however, the agency chose to specify that the conditional-sail order would be automatically rescinded upon "expiration" of the PHE determination (CDC, 2022a). This choice was consistent with the agency's discretionary reliance on the PHE determination to determine how long its order would meet the statutory standard of "necessity" under Section 361(a).

---

[14] CDC, *Requirement for Airlines and Operators to Collect and Transmit Designated Information for Passengers and Crew Arriving into the U.S.; Requirement for Passengers to Provide Designated Information* (October 25, 2021).

[15] This text was modified after release of the report to the study sponsor to correctly represent isolation orders made by the CDC.

[16] CDC, *No Sail Order and Other Measures Related to Operations* (March 14, 2020). 85 FR 16628.

[17] CDC, Framework for Conditional Sailing Order (October 30, 2020). 85 FR 70153.

> **BOX 6-1**
> **Proposed Quarantining of Diamond Cruise Ship Passengers**
>
> In February 2020, an outbreak of COVID-19 occurred on a *Diamond Princess* cruise ship, infecting over 600 passengers and resulting in three deaths. Approximately 300 American passengers—14 of whom tested positive for COVID-19—were evacuated from the ship by the U.S. government. On February 22, 2020, the Department of Health and Human Services (HHS) announced a plan to quarantine these American passengers in a Federal Emergency Management Agency (FEMA) center in Anniston, Alabama. The mayor and other local leaders in Anniston voiced concerns, including lack of preparation and notice, not being given the opportunity to provide input, the speed involved in the federal government's decision, and their lack of knowledge of the plan's details, such as which hospitals HHS had "pre-identified" as designated care facilities.
>
> On February 23, 2020, the Anniston County City Council approved a resolution to pursue legal action against the federal government to prevent passengers from being transferred to the county for quarantine. While most officials and residents voiced support for the measure, Council Member Jay Jenkins emphasized that the passengers were Americans in need of help and health care. Alabama Governor Kay Ivey, Senator Richard Shelby, and U.S. Representative Mike Rogers announced on social media that they received assurances from President Donald Trump that no *Diamond Princess* passengers would be transferred to Anniston. The White House did not comment on the decision to abandon the plan.
>
> Simultaneously, a similar series of events played out in Costa Mesa, California, after the federal government designated a vacated, state-owned facility that once housed residents with developmental disabilities as an isolation site for passengers from the *Diamond Princess* cruise ship who tested positive for COVID-19. Local officials objected, stating that they were not included in the planning process and citing concerns for the safety of Costa Mesa residents. On February 21, 2020, U.S. District Judge Josephine Stanton in Costa Mesa issued a restraining order that blocked the federal government from transferring the passengers to the city. On February 28, 2020, the federal government announced that the plan to isolate passengers in Costa Mesa had been abandoned.
>
> SOURCES: Associated Press, 2020; Canales, 2020; Pereira, 2020; Whitcomb, 2020.

Border Control

On March 20, 2020, the CDC issued an order suspending crossings at U.S. land borders by "persons traveling from Canada or Mexico (regardless of their country of origin) who would otherwise be introduced into a congregate setting in a land Port of Entry (POE) or Border Patrol station."[18] The order emphasized crowded conditions at immigration processing fa-

---

[18] CDC, Order Suspending Introduction of Certain Persons from Countries Where a Communicable Disease Exists (March 20, 2020).

cilities, which are "not equipped to quarantine, isolate, or enable social distancing."[19] Under the order, which has been periodically renewed by the Trump and Biden administrations and remains in effect as of this writing, U.S. border authorities have relied on what has become known as the "Title 42 process"—named for the title of the U.S. Code where the PHSA is codified—to expel nearly 1.5 million migrants without screening them to determine whether they qualify for asylum (Montoya-Galvez, 2022). Because the CDC lacks implementation capacity, the border crossing order is implemented by CBP pursuant to a request from the CDC director to the Department of Homeland Security (DHS) and at the direction of the president. The order references "public health emergency" conditions generally, but it does not include an automatic rescission provision tethered to rescission of the HHS secretary's Section 319 determination.

Residential Eviction Moratorium Orders

On September 4, 2020, following initial congressional authority, the CDC issued an order strictly regulating residential evictions for nonpayment of rent.[20] The order applied to tenants who met income eligibility criteria and had exhausted available means of obtaining assistance. To establish the nexus with the interstate spread of disease, the order required tenants to provide a declaration under penalty of perjury that they would likely be homeless or forced to move into a congregate or shared living situation if evicted. The order relied on PHSA Section 361(a) (CDC, 2021a; Congressional Research Service, 2021a).

The CDC supported the order with data showing the effect of homelessness on the spread of infectious diseases. Congress first initiated the order under the CARES Act from March 2020 to July 2020. Once expired, the CDC's eviction moratorium took effect on September 4, 2020, and was extended periodically until June 30, 2021 (Congressional Research Service, 2021a). After the CDC allowed its standing eviction moratorium to lapse and in response to litigation threatening to block the moratorium on the grounds that it exceeded its authority, the CDC issued a new order on August 3, 2021, limited to counties meeting the CDC's thresholds for substantial or high rates of community transmission.[21] The eviction mora-

---

[19] Id.

[20] The initial CDC order was issued shortly after a prior eviction moratorium instituted by Congress under Section 4024 of the CARES Act had expired, but the CDC moratorium was broader than the legislative one, which applied only to tenants receiving federal rental assistance.

[21] CDC, Temporary Halt in Residential Evictions in Communities with Substantial or High Transmission of COVID-19 To Prevent the Further Spread of COVID-19, 86 Fed. Reg. 43244 (August 6, 2021).

torium orders did not include an automatic rescission provision tethered to rescission of the HHS secretary's PHE determination. The CDC eviction moratoria went well beyond its previous orders, as it focused on housing and homelessness and was struck down by the U.S. Supreme Court despite previously allowing the moratorium to stand just weeks earlier.[22]

Transit Face-Mask Order

Under PHSA Section 361(a), on January 29, 2021, the CDC issued an order requiring workers and passengers to wear face masks on shared conveyances and in transportation hubs. In addition to Section 361, the order referenced the CDC's regulations relating to carriers.[23] To establish the order's nexus to interstate and international commerce and travel, the CDC emphasized that "intrastate transmission of the virus has led to—and continues to lead to—interstate and international spread of the virus, particularly on public conveyances and in travel hubs, where passengers who may themselves be traveling only within their state or territory commonly interact with others traveling between states or territories or internationally."[24] The Transportation Security Administration (TSA) issued a security directive to enforce the CDC's order.

The TSA's Security Directive was periodically renewed and was set to expire on May 3, 2022. But on April 18, a federal judge in the Middle District of Florida issued a nationwide injunction against enforcement of the transit mask requirement. The TSA immediately stopped enforcement of the order. While the CDC did not indicate it would reinstitute the mask order at the time, it informed the Department of Justice (DOJ) that having the power to order mask use was still "necessary." At the time of writing, the DOJ had filed an appeal against the judge's ruling to the U.S. Court of Appeals for the 11th Circuit. The DOJ did not seek an emergency stay of the judge's nationwide injunction (Gostin and Hosie, 2022).

The CDC's transit mask order was enforced by the TSA and other federal transit agencies and "may be enforced by cooperating state and local authorities."[25] The CDC does not have authority to direct the TSA to enforce its orders, but the president has the authority to coordinate the actions of federal agencies. President Biden signed an executive order on January 21, 2021, directing the HHS secretary, the TSA, and "any other executive . . . agencies . . . that have relevant regulatory authority" to take action,

---

[22] 141 S. Ct. 2320 (2021).
[23] 42 CFR §71.31(b) and 71.32(b).
[24] CDC, Requirement for Persons to Wear Masks While on Conveyances and at Transportation Hubs, 86 Fed. Reg. 8025 (January 29, 2021).
[25] Id.

"to the extent appropriate and consistent with applicable law, to require masks to be worn in compliance with CDC guidelines" in airports and on public transportation.[26] The DHS responded by issuing an emergency determination indicating that TSA will support the CDC "in the enforcement of any orders or other requirements necessary to protect the transportation system...."[27] The TSA then issued a series of security directives to enforce the CDC's order.[28]

The CDC's transit mask order includes an automatic rescission provision tethered to the HHS secretary's PHE determination. As for the cruise conditional-sail order, this choice was not mandated by statute, but is consistent with the CDC's discretionary reliance on a PHE determination in determining how long its order would meet the "necessity" standard under Section 361(a).

Predeparture Testing Requirements for Air Passengers Entering the United States and Vaccination Requirements under Immigration Authorities

On December 25, 2020, the CDC issued an order requiring airlines to ensure that all passengers aged two and older (including U.S. citizens) arriving in the United States from the United Kingdom submit predeparture test results (U.S. Embassy & Consulates in the United Kingdom, 2021). This order was issued in the context of reports that the more transmissible SARS-CoV-2 alpha variant was widely circulating in the United Kingdom. On January 12, 2021, the CDC issued a new order requiring predeparture testing for all airline passengers aged two and older arriving from any foreign country (CDC, 2022c). The later order, which has been periodically renewed and remains in effect as of this writing, allows an exemption for passengers who provide documentation of recent infection. In addition to referring to PHSA Section 361(a), these orders referenced the CDC's regulations relating to "public health prevention measures, at U.S.[29] ports of entry or other locations, through noninvasive procedures . . . to detect the potential presence of communicable disease" and issuance of "controlled free pratique" stipulating conditions for carriers' entry, disembarkation, or

---

[26] Executive Order 13998, 86 Fed. Reg. 7205 (January 21, 2021).

[27] DHS, Determination of a National Emergency Requiring Actions to Protect the Safety of Americans Using and Employed by the Transportation System (DHS Determination 21-130) (January 27, 2021).

[28] TSA, Security Measures—Mask Requirements (TSA Security Directive 1582/84-21-01) (January 31, 2021).

[29] 42 CFR §71.20.

operation in certain stipulated conditions.[30] These orders also include an automatic rescission provision tethered to the PHE determination.

On October 25, 2021, President Biden issued an order rescinding country-specific prohibitions on entry into the United States and replacing them with a directive that noncitizen nonimmigrants entering the United States by air must provide proof of vaccination for COVID-19.[31] The presidential order relies on the president's immigration powers, not the CDC's powers. Thus, the order does not apply to U.S. citizens.[32]

Court Rulings on COVID-19 Relying on Narrow Interpretation of the Public Health Service Act

Recent court rulings have interpreted the PHSA narrowly. In 2021, the Supreme Court and lower federal courts enjoined the CDC's eviction moratorium order in *Alabama Association of Realtors v. Department of Health and Human Services*. The same year, a federal district court judge enjoined the CDC's cruise conditional-sail order and a circuit court panel declined to postpone implementation of the injunction in *Florida v. Becerra*. Also in 2021, a federal district court judge enjoined the CDC's border control order, but a circuit court panel postponed implementation of the injunction in *Huisha-Huisha v. Mayorkas*. Additionally, a suit challenging the CDC's transit mask order is pending in federal district court.

Enjoinment of the CDC's Eviction Moratorium Order

In *Alabama Association of Realtors v. Department of Health and Human Services*, the U.S. Supreme Court enjoined the CDC's eviction moratorium order, holding that the plaintiffs were substantially likely to succeed on their claim that the order exceeded the CDC's statutory authority. The Supreme Court's ruling followed a series of lower court rulings, in which most courts determined that the CDC had exceeded its statutory authority.[33] The Supreme Court majority based its decision on statutory

---

[30] 42 CFR §71.31(b).

[31] Proclamation 10294, Advancing the Safe Resumption of Global Travel During the COVID-19 Pandemic, 86 Fed. Reg. 206 (Oct. 25, 2021).

[32] This paragraph was modified after release of the report to the study sponsor to clarify the type of entrant and mode of travel covered by this presidential order.

[33] See, e.g., *Tiger Lily, LLC v. Dep't of Housing & Urban Dev.*, 5 F.4th 666 (6th Cir. 2021) (holding eviction order exceeded CDC's statutory authority); *Terkel v. Ctrs. for Disease Control & Prevention*, 521 F. Supp. 3d 662 (E.D. Tex. 2021) (accord); *Skyworks, Ltd. v. Ctrs. for Disease Control & Prevention*, 524 F.Supp.3d 745 (N.D. Ohio 2021) (accord); but see *Chambliss Enterprises v. Redfield*, 508 F.Supp.3d 101 (W.D. La. 2020) (holding CDC's eviction order did not exceed its statutory authority).

interpretation alone, without resorting to constitutional arguments that would constrain Congress's ability to empower the CDC to regulate residential evictions in more specific terms. The Court reasoned that the second sentence of Section 361(a), which lists specific examples of how the CDC may use its power, "informs the grant of authority" in the first sentence.[34] The Court described the examples listed in the second sentence as measures that "*directly relate* to preventing the interstate spread of disease by identifying, isolating, and destroying the disease itself."[35] In contrast, the court determined the eviction moratorium "relates to interstate infection far more indirectly: If evictions occur, some subset of tenants might move from one State to another, and some subset of that group might do so while infected with COVID-19."[36] Thus, the court concluded the CDC order should be enjoined pending appeal because "reading both sentences together, rather than the first in isolation, it is a stretch to maintain that §361(a) gives the CDC the authority to impose this eviction moratorium."[37]

Enjoinment of the CDC's Cruise Conditional-Sail Order

In *Florida v. Becerra*, a federal district court judge granted Florida's request for a preliminary injunction blocking the CDC from enforcing its cruise ship conditional-sail order.[38] The judge held that the state was likely to succeed on the merits of its claims because—among other arguments discussed in the following—the order exceeded the CDC's authority. The Eleventh Circuit initially stayed the district court's order, postponing implementation of the injunction and permitting the CDC to enforce the cruise ship order while litigation continued. A week later, shortly after Florida filed a petition asking the Supreme Court to intervene in the case, the Eleventh Circuit reversed this ruling, effectively blocking CDC enforcement. Thus far, the Eleventh Circuit's decision appears to have dissuaded the Supreme Court from intervening in the litigation (which continues).

The district court's opinion determined that the second sentence of Section 361(a) (listing specific examples) "operates to limit CDC's enforcement and implementation authority to *only those actions resembling* 'inspection, fumigation, disinfection, ... [and] pest extermination.'"[39] The court described the cruise ship orders as "halting commerce by a fifteen-month closure of one or more industries" and determined that action was not "similar in scope and character the measures contemplated and autho-

---

[34] Ala. Ass'n of Realtors, 141 S.Ct. at 2488.
[35] Id. (emphasis added).
[36] Id.
[37] Id.
[38] *Florida v. Becerra*, 544 F.Supp.3d 1241 (M.D. Fla. 2021).
[39] Id. at 1268.

rized by Congress when enacting the statute."⁴⁰ In dicta, the judge opined that "halting other public movement and activity nationwide" would also exceed the CDC's authority.⁴¹ To support his reading, the judge reasoned that prior to the COVID-19 pandemic, federal health officials had deployed measures that "resemble" the examples specifically enumerated in Section 361(a) but had not done anything resembling "the conditional sailing order's mandates."⁴²

Enjoinment of the CDC's Border-Control Order

In *Huisha-Huisha v. Mayorkas*, a federal district court judge granted the plaintiff class's request for a preliminary injunction blocking the administration from relying on the CDC's Section 362 authority to expel migrants. The judge reasoned that Section 362, which allows the CDC to suspend introduction of persons into the United States "simply contains no mention of the word "expel"—or any synonyms thereof—within its text." Consistent with what the Supreme Court has called the "major questions doctrine," the judge reasoned that courts "expect Congress to speak clearly if it wishes to assign to an agency decisions of vast 'economic and political significance,'" ⁴³ the judge ruled that the CDC had exceeded its authority. A three-judge panel of the DC Circuit granted the Biden administration's request to stay the district court's injunction while their appeal is pending.⁴⁴ As of this writing, the appeal is under review and the administration continues to enforce the order.

Pending Suit Challenging the CDC's Transit Mask Order

The CDC's transit mask order has also been challenged in lawsuits filed in 2021 by private parties in the Middle District of Florida⁴⁵ and a new suit filed in February 2022 by the state of Texas (joined by a private plaintiff) in the Eastern District of Texas.⁴⁶ The judges assigned to hear these cases

---

⁴⁰ Id.
⁴¹ Id.
⁴² Id. at 1269.
⁴³ *Huisha-Huisha v. Mayorkas*, __F.Supp.3d.__, 2021 WL 4206688, *11 (D.D.C. 2021).
⁴⁴ *Huisha-Huisha v. Mayorkas*, Civ. No. 1:21-cv-00100-EGS (D.C. Cir., September 30, 2021) (granting motion for a stay pending appeal).
⁴⁵ *Health Freedom Def. Fund v. Biden*, Civ No. 8:21-cv-1693-KKM-AEP (M.D. Fla., November 19, 2021) (denying defendant's motion to transfer action to another judge hearing a similar challenge); *Wall v. Ctrs. for Disease Control*, Case No: 6:21-cv-975-PGB-DCI (M.D. Fla, December 18, 2021) (dismissing claims on procedural grounds without prejudice and thus allowing the plaintiff to refile in the future).
⁴⁶ *Van Duyne v. Ctrs. for Disease Control*, Case No. 4:22-cv-00122-O (N.D. Tex.) (complaint filed February 16, 2022).

have not yet opined on the merits of the plaintiffs' challenges, but the order could be vulnerable under a narrow reading of Section 361(a) given that the statute does not specifically endorse orders mandating the use of PPE. Alternatively, the judges could find that the transit mask order "directly relate[s] to preventing the interstate spread of disease by . . . isolating . . . the disease itself" (the Supreme Court's formulation in *Alabama Association of Realtors*) and thus is similar enough to the examples specified in Section 361(a) to fall within the CDC's authority.

Taking all these, and other, cases as a whole, it is apparent to the committee that the CDC interventions to stem the introduction to or spread of disease within the United States have often been delayed or blocked by the courts. This underscores the need for legislative and regulatory reform to ensure the CDC can exercise needed authority to protect the American population.

MODERNIZING THE CDC'S PANDEMIC PREVENTION AND RESPONSE AUTHORITY

The committee concludes that reforms are needed to modernize the CDC'S pandemic prevention and response powers and to provide appropriate substantive and procedural safeguards of individual liberties. In the wake of recent court decisions, there is considerable uncertainty about the extent of the CDC's power to implement measures that are not specifically listed as examples in the PHSA. Uncertainty about the scope of the CDC's authority is particularly concerning given the limitations of other government actors. It is also concerning because the CDC must be able to act decisively and lawfully in a public health crisis.

State, tribal, local, and territorial (STLT) entities lack comprehensive authority over international and interstate commerce and travel. Congress lacks capacity for the swift responses and nimble adjustments required to prevent or manage a pandemic. The courts could interpret the Supreme Court's opinion in *Alabama Association of Realtors* to permit the CDC to require face coverings, proof of a negative test, self-quarantine on arrival, or proof of vaccination on interstate conveyances and in transit hubs. However, additional clarification from the courts may not be forthcoming.

Harmonization of STLT efforts is necessary for best use of regulatory authority and infectious disease mitigation. As highlighted in the "Improving Coordination and Collaboration to Enhance Disease Control" chapter conclusions, including federal interagency partners and interstate relationships in coordination efforts could provide the CDC with greater opportunities to best support state jurisdictions effectively.

To mitigate the chilling effect of uncertainty and incorporate lessons learned from the COVID-19 pandemic, the committee recommends that

Congress modernize the CDC's pandemic prevention and response powers. In addition, regardless of whether Congress amends Section 361, we recommend that the CDC initiate rulemaking to clarify its interpretation of the broadly delineated "necessary measures" provision and adopt procedural requirements and substantive standards to govern the use of its powers. Our recommended reforms will need to be consistent with constitutional limits and must ensure the CDC's powers are comprehensive, effective, flexible, and exercised in ways that are consistent with principles of good governance and equity.

Constitutional and Statutory Limits on Expansion of the CDC's Authority

Reforms to modernize the PHSA must be consistent with constitutional and statutory limits on expansion of the CDC's authority, namely: federalism limits, separation of powers and administrative law limits, and protections for individual rights. The balance the committee is seeking is to ensure prompt exercise of all powers needed to protect the public from the introduction or spread of infectious diseases, while ensuring that the CDC acts according to the available scientific evidence and consistent with the protection of individual rights. The committee also wishes to ensure that CDC powers are exercised fairly and equitably.

Federalism Limits

The powers that Congress delegates to the CDC must fall within the limited federal powers enumerated in the Constitution, including the power to regulate interstate commerce and travel, the power to attach conditions to federal spending, and various foreign policy powers, including treaties. If the spread of a communicable disease is confined to a single state—and likely to remain so—then the federal government's regulatory power is far more limited. Federal influence can be expanded by constitutionally conditioning acceptance of federal funds on adoption of specific public health measures. However, spending conditions would not readily enable the flexible powers the CDC needs for pandemic prevention and response.

Separation of Powers and Administrative Law Limits

Some lower federal courts have gone further than the Supreme Court majority by basing their decisions enjoining the CDC's orders on constitutional constraints that limit Congress's ability to delegate authority to the CDC in broadly delineated terms. For example, in *Tiger Lily, LLC*, the Sixth Circuit reasoned that the CDC's broad interpretation of Section 361(a) should be rejected under the major questions doctrine, which holds that "Congress must 'enact exceedingly clear language if it wishes to significantly alter the balance between federal and state power and the power of the Government over private property.'"[47] In addition, the Sixth Circuit suggested the CDC's broad interpretation of Section 361(a)'s "other measures" language "could raise a nondelegation problem (Congressional Research Service, 2021b)" The nondelegation doctrine holds that Congress is constitutionally prohibited from delegating authority to the executive branch in "open-ended" terms that do not provide sufficient standards to limit agency discretion over policy choices. The Sixth Circuit explicitly rejected the CDC's argument that public health necessity provided a sufficient standard to guide the agency's exercise of discretion. Similarly, in *Florida v. Becerra*, the federal district court judge reasoned that if Congress had intended to give the CDC such broad authority under Section 361(a), it would amount to an unconstitutional delegation of legislative power. This reasoning informed his narrow interpretation of the statute's language, based on the principle that judges should endeavor to construe statutes in ways that avoid rendering them unconstitutional.

The doctrines endorsed by some lower court judges in the eviction moratorium and cruise conditional-sail cases are highly controversial. Legal scholars have pointed out that they have not yet won the support of a majority of the Supreme Court, but that could change in the near future. Such a change "would mark a radical break with constitutional practice and could entail the wholesale repudiation of modern American governance" (Mortenson and Bagley, 2021, p.278). It would have particularly devastating consequences for pandemic prevention and response capabilities, given how legislatures have traditionally relied on broadly delineated delegations of authority to health agencies to control communicable diseases using measures consistent with public health necessity.

Reforms should also require the CDC to follow appropriate procedures to ensure its orders are promulgated transparently and through processes that foster the public's trust and cooperation. The Administrative Procedure Act (APA), Congressional Review Act (CRA), and other statutes set forth procedures that agencies must follow when they issue rules. In *Florida v. Becerra*, the federal district court judge determined that CDC's cruise conditional-sail order was a "rule" within the meaning of the APA and, therefore, the state was likely to succeed on its claim that the CDC had failed to follow required notice and comment procedures. The Government Accountability Office (GAO) has opined that the CDC's transit mask order is a "rule" for the purposes of the CRA and that the CDC violated the CRA

---

[47] Quotation from another decision. *U.S. Forest Serv. v. Cowpasture River Pres. Ass'n*, 140 S. Ct. 1837, 1849–1850 (2020).

by failing to submit it for congressional review.[48] Similar claims have been raised against the CDC's other orders, but the Supreme Court has not yet reached these questions.

The procedures that govern the CDC's exercise of its authority under Section 361(a) and Section 362 are not detailed in the statute or accompanying regulations. In some of its COVID-19 orders, the CDC asserted that the order was not a "rule" subject to the APA's notice and comment requirements, and, in the alternative, if it were a rule, then the APA's "good cause" exception applied.[49] But lower court decisions indicate that in the future, the CDC may need to engage in more formal procedures. New legislation or CDC rulemaking should set forth these procedures more clearly.

Protections for Individual Rights

It will be critical that the CDC's actions respect constitutional and statutory protections for individual rights. To date, the CDC's COVID-19 orders have not been successfully challenged on these grounds. Were the CDC to limit gatherings or restrict gathering places, businesses, or travel in the future, court decisions reviewing state and local COVID-19 orders would provide useful guidance. The First Amendment's Free Exercise and Establishment Clauses and the federal and state Religious Freedom Restoration Acts protect religious liberty. Under the new Supreme Court majority's emerging jurisprudence, if a CDC order includes any secular exemption, the lack of a religious exemption on equal or better terms may trigger strict scrutiny by the courts.[50] First Amendment protections for freedom of expression and assembly may limit the extent to which gathering limits restrict political events or protests.[51] The Second Amendment's protection for the

---

[48] GAO, Centers for Disease Control & Prevention—Applicability of Congressional Review Act to Requirement for Persons to Wear Masks While on Conveyances and at Transportation Hubs (December 14, 2021).

[49] 5 U.S.C. §553(b)(3)(B).

[50] See, e.g., *Tandon v. Newsom*, 141 S.Ct. 1294 (2021) (barring California officials from enforcing generally applicable gathering restrictions against religious gatherings, including in private homes); but see *Does 1-3 v. Mills*, 142 S.Ct.17 (2021) (denying an application for injunctive relief and thus allowing Maine officials to implement a vaccination requirement for health care workers that allowed medical exemptions, but not religious exemptions).

[51] The lower courts have applied more deferential (rational basis) review to restrictions on social gatherings compared to the heightened or strict scrutiny some have applied to restrictions on gatherings for religious or political purposes. See *Henry v. DeSantis*, 461 F.Supp.3d 1244, 1254 (S.D. Fla. 2020) (denying a request for preliminary injunction for a plaintiff who did not have any specific plans to engage in political protests after finding no "generalized right of *social* association under the First Amendment's freedom of association").

right to bear arms may constrain restrictions that affect firearm purchases.[52] The extent to which the Constitution protects freedom of movement and travel during PHEs is uncertain. At least one lower court closely scrutinized a state order requiring interstate travelers to self-quarantine, but found the requirement satisfied the strict scrutiny standard because a less restrictive alternative was not reasonably available at the time.[53] Privacy protections apply to the CDC's collection, storage, and use of personal health information. The Health Insurance Portability and Accountability Act (HIPAA) Privacy Rule does not govern the CDC's actions, and exceptions to the Privacy Rule allow covered entities to share protected health information with the CDC or other federal or STLT public health authorities.[54] The CDC is governed by the Privacy Act of 1974[55] and the Confidential Information Protection and Statistical Efficiency Act of 2002,[56] which establish data security and confidentiality requirements for personally identifiable information collected and stored by federal agencies.

Clarifying the Scope and Limits of the CDC's Authority

We recommend that Congress modernize the PHSA to clarify the scope and limits of the CDC's authority when narrowly targeted containment measures fail. To fill gaps in STLT powers and ensure capacity for a nationally coordinated response to prevent and mitigate future pandemics, we recommend that Congress amend the PHSA to specify that the "necessary measures" authorized in Section 361(a) may include regulation of international and interstate travel, requirements to wear face coverings or other PPE, restrictions on mass gatherings, occupancy limits or sanitation requirements for gathering places, protections to support compliance with public

---

[52] See, e.g., *McDougall v. County of Ventura*, Civ. No. 20-56220 (9th Cir. January 20, 2022) (holding that COVID-19 orders closing gun shops failed strict scrutiny and, in the alternative, failed intermediate scrutiny); *but see Dark Storm Industries LLC v. Cuomo*, 471 F.Supp.3d 482 (N.D.N.Y 2020) (granting summary judgment against plaintiffs after applying intermediate scrutiny to their claim alleging governor's order closing gun shops violated their Second Amendment rights) (judgment vacated and appeal dismissed as moot on October 5, 2021).

[53] *Bayley's Campground, Inc. v. Mills*, 958 F.3d 153 (2021) (assuming, without deciding, that strict scrutiny was the proper standard for reviewing Maine's executive order requiring interstate travelers to self-quarantine on arrival and prohibiting them from doing so in temporary lodgings within the state, but finding strict scrutiny was probably satisfied because no less restrictive alternative was reasonably available at a time when COVID-19 testing was not readily accessible). Other courts applying more deferential standards to self-quarantine requirements for interstate travelers relied on an interpretation of *Jacobson v. Massachusetts* that the Supreme Court has indicated it disfavors.

[54] 45 CFR §164.512(b).

[55] 5 U.S.C. §552a.

[56] 44 U.S.C. §3501 et seq.

health guidance, as well as other necessary powers. As for the measures specified in Section 361(a)–(d), use of these powers would be contingent on a finding by the CDC director that they "are necessary to prevent the introduction, transmission, or spread of communicable diseases from foreign countries into the States or possessions, or from one State or possession into any other State or possession."[57] The COVID-19 pandemic has revealed how a coordinated, evidence-based national strategy is needed to prevent and control dangerous infectious disease outbreaks. The CDC ought to have ample powers to do that, consistent with the federal government's constitutional obligations to prevent hazards in interstate or international commerce and act expressly in the interests of national security.

It is also important to ensure that the CDC does not overreach or exceed its legitimate regulatory authority. PHSA amendments will need to specify the conditions that must be met before the CDC may use its Section 361(a) powers to mandate protections that apply to the general public regardless of known or suspected infection or exposure. A particularly apt guardrail that the CDC voluntarily adopted for some, but not all, of its COVID-19 orders was an automatic rescission provision tethering the continued necessity of the CDC's order under Section 361(a) to the termination of the HHS secretary's PHE determination under Section 319. The current text of the PHSA does not condition any of the CDC's powers on the existence of a PHE. Some uses of Section 361(a) powers—such as the CDC's isolation of an individual traveler reasonably believed to be infected with extensively drug-resistant tuberculosis or the Food and Drug Administration's (FDA) prohibition on the sale of pet turtles that may carry salmonella[58]—should not be conditioned on a PHE. But intrusive or disruptive measures applied to the general public in the absence of individualized risk assessments to determine known or suspected infection or exposure should be contingent on the HHS secretary's PHE determination and additional criteria by which the HHS secretary may determine that more narrowly targeted interventions are insufficient to prevent the interstate spread of disease.

We recommend that Congress amend the PHSA to add a new subsection. The new subsection would parallel Sections 361(b)–(d), which set forth the conditions under which Section 361(a) powers may be used to apprehend, detain, or conditionally release individuals. Drawing on language used in other subsections, our proposed new Section 361(f) would be as follows:

---

[57] 42 U.S. Code §264.
[58] *Independent Turtle Farmers of Louisiana, Inc. v. U.S.*, 703 F.Supp.2d 604 (W.D. La. 2010) (upholding an FDA ban on sale of small turtles under Section 361). Like the CDC, the FDA has powers under Section 361(a) thanks to a delegation of authority from the HHS secretary.

Regulations prescribed under this section may provide for restrictions on or requirements for persons engaged in international or interstate travel, requirements to wear face coverings or other personal protective equipment in specified settings, restrictions on mass gatherings, occupancy limits or sanitation requirements for gathering places, and protections related to housing and employment for the purpose of supporting compliance with public health guidance. These measures may be prescribed in the absence of individualized risk assessments only upon a determination by the HHS secretary that:

(1) a public health emergency exists as set forth in section 247d(a) of this title;
(2) apprehension, detention, examination, and conditional release of individuals based on known or reasonably suspected infection or exposure and inspection, fumigation, disinfection, sanitation, pest extermination, or destruction of animals or articles found to be infected or contaminated would not be effective in preventing the introduction, transmission, or spread of a designated list of communicable diseases from foreign countries into the States or possessions, or from one State or possession into any other State or possession; and
(3) STLT regulations are insufficient to prevent the introduction, transmission, or spread of communicable diseases from foreign countries into the States or possessions, or from one State or possession into any other State or possession.

This language would provide the specificity some federal judges require while also imposing appropriate limits that are not currently mandated by statute. Key terms (e.g. "gatherings" and "gathering places") would be left for the CDC to define via rulemaking.

We recommend that Congress preserve the language in Section 361(a) authorizing "other measures" officials deem necessary. A future threat could pose unforeseen dangers or require measures that lawmakers cannot anticipate in specific terms. In such a scenario, the courts may be more forgiving of the CDC's use of broadly delineated powers than they have been during the COVID-19 pandemic. One approach would be to amend Section 361(e) to add a savings clause expressly stating: "Regulations prescribed under this section shall not preempt state and local regulations that are more protective of public health."

We recommend that the CDC's exercise of Section 361 powers establish a federal floor of public health protection without preempting state and local governments from adopting evidence-based additional layers of protection. Were the issue to be litigated—and to date it has not been—courts may interpret the current language in Section 361(e) to spare more stringent state and local laws from federal preemption. However, Congress could speak even more clearly on this issue to prevent federal officials from using Section 361 powers to prohibit state and local public health protections.

For some measures adopted in some settings, federal resources for implementation and enforcement are likely to be inadequate—even when the president directs other federal agencies to assist. But a CDC order that creates a floor of protections by preempting conflicting state laws could empower local governments to implement and enforce public health protections using their own resources, without interference from state governments who oppose them.

Rulemaking to Clarify the Scope and Limits of the CDC's Powers Under Section 361(a)

We recommend that the CDC initiate rulemaking to clarify the scope and limits of its powers under Section 361(a). Whether or not Congress amends Section 361, the CDC should adopt definitions, procedural requirements, and substantive standards to govern orders that are not based on known or suspected infection or exposure of specific individuals. In a multiyear process completed in 2017, the CDC modernized its regulations for interstate and international quarantine and isolation of individuals. The 2017 rules adopt significant protections to ensure the CDC's quarantine, isolation, and conditional release orders are consistent with the best available scientific evidence and constitutional protections. But these reforms failed to address the scope and limits of the CDC's authority to mitigate widespread community transmission when targeted containment efforts fail.

New regulations applicable to the CDC's use of its powers under the "necessary measures" provision in Section 361(a) would guide officials when they exercise discretion under existing (or newly amended) statutory authorities. However, such regulatory reforms may not overcome narrow statutory interpretations by the federal courts.

SURGE FUNDING FOR OUTBREAK RESPONSE

Challenges in Obtaining Timely Surge Funding

Historically, funding for large-scale public health emergencies has primarily relied on redirecting (i.e., reprogramming) appropriated funds from other day-to-day mission requirements, generally from HHS annual budgets (Alton and Carlin, 2020). During certain infectious disease outbreaks—such as the H1N1 influenza pandemic (2009), the Ebola virus disease epidemic (2014–2016), the Zika virus disease outbreak (2015–2016), and the COVID-19 pandemic—Congress passed supplemental appropriations to fund response activities. However, the surge funding often came late, and these congressional actions were often politically controversial.

The Public Health Emergency Fund (PHEF),[59] established in 1983, is available to the secretary of HHS without fiscal year limitation to take appropriate action in response to a public health emergency.[60] Apart from special congressional appropriations from the PHEF during a PHE,[61] reserve funds for outbreak response primarily come from HHS and its various operating divisions (Alton and Carlin, 2020). In responding to the 2009 H1N1 influenza pandemic, multiple HHS programs "assessed" funds to be reprogrammed, as allowed by statute, to cover costs for development and production of the vaccine. This maneuver adversely impacted multiple programs for many years. For instance, the Strategic National Stockpile[62] (SNS) had programmed funds to obligate to a vaccine contract to the Chemical, Biological, Radiological and Nuclear Office (CBRN) that were lost to funding for the H1N1 event and never replaced (Congressional Research Service, 2009; Simon and Evstatieva, 2020). This initiated a shortfall in medical countermeasures for CBRN events that continues today (Burel, 2020). Similarly, in an effort to respond to the Zika crisis (2015–2016), the CDC had to move funds from critical programs to cover costs that were immediately required (Boddie, 2015; DeLauro, n.d.). During the Ebola epidemic (2014–2016), the SNS had to move money planned for purchasing medical countermeasures for CBRN emergency response, resulting in shortfalls in other critical material needs (Boddie, 2015; DeLauro, n.d.).

---

[59] "There is established in the Treasury a fund to be designated as the "Public Health Emergency Fund" to be made available to the secretary without fiscal year limitation to carry out subsection (a) only if a public health emergency has been declared by the secretary under such subsection or if the secretary determines there is the significant potential for a public health emergency, to allow the secretary to rapidly respond to the immediate needs resulting from such public health emergency or potential public health emergency. The secretary shall plan for the expedited distribution of funds to appropriate agencies and entities. There is authorized to be appropriated to the Fund such sums as may be necessary . . ." Public Health Emergencies, 42 U.S. Code §247d. (1983).

[60] See Pub. L. No. 98-49, 97 Stat. 245 (1983).

[61] "If the secretary determines, after consultation with such public health officials as may be necessary, that—(1) a disease or disorder presents a public health emergency; or (2) a public health emergency, including significant outbreaks of infectious diseases or bioterrorist attacks, otherwise exists, the secretary may take such action as may be appropriate to respond to the public health emergency, including making grants, providing awards for expenses, and entering into contracts and conducting and supporting investigations into the cause, treatment, or prevention of a disease or disorder . . ." Public Health Emergencies, 42 U.S. Code §247d. (1983) (Source: https://www.law.cornell.edu/uscode/text/42/247d; accessed March 4, 2022).

[62] The Strategic National Stockpile, within the Office of the Assistant Secretary for Preparedness and Response, is "part of the federal medical response infrastructure and can supplement medical countermeasures needed by states, tribal nations, territories and the largest metropolitan areas during public health emergencies." More information is available from https://www.phe.gov/about/sns/Pages/default.aspx (accessed March 4, 2022).

The mere existence of federal mechanisms to mobilize assistance to state and local governments does not guarantee adequate and timely funding during an outbreak (Katz et al., 2017). For instance, political contentions can delay passage of emergency appropriations legislation acceptable to both Congress and the White House. Likewise, Congress took a full year to authorize President Obama's emergency funding request for the Zika response (Gostin, 2018). Funding for the Ebola response was delayed for months (NACCHO, 2017). Congress did not appropriate funding for the Ebola response until December 2014, even though the federal, state, and local public health response had been ongoing since summer 2014 and the first case in the United States was confirmed that September.

These challenges underscore the extent to which the current method of emergency response funding from committed appropriations is neither suitable nor sufficient. Reliance on supplemental appropriations for every discrete response raises the possibilities that Congress (1) may choose not to approve funds (DeBonis, 2021), (2) will approve inadequate funds (O'Toole, 2007), (3) will direct funding in particular directions which do not align with public health priorities, and (4) will act too slowly to contain contagious disease (DeLauro, n.d.).

Ways to Streamline Mechanisms for Surge Funding

The Committee considered a range of opportunities to streamline and expedite surge funding mechanisms by mitigating the challenges inherent in the current structure. Proposed alternatives include:

- Establishing a new public health emergency contingency fund that can be triggered under certain criteria during a public health emergency,
- Establishing a fund similar to the HHS's Federal Emergency Management Agency's (FEMA) Disaster Relief Fund (DRF) (FEMA, 2013), or
- Appropriating funds to the existing enacted Public Health Emergency Fund that has not received appropriations since FY1999, with the account maintaining a zero balance since 2012 (Katz et al., 2017), and
- Appropriating funds to the proposed Infectious Disease Rapid Response Reserve Fund[63] (Alton and Carlin, 2020).

---

[63] "There is established in the Treasury a reserve fund to be known as the "Infectious Diseases Rapid Response Reserve Fund" (the "Reserve Fund"): Provided, That of the funds provided under the heading "CDC-Wide Activities and Program Support" [132 Stat. 3073], $50,000,000, to remain available until expended, shall be available to the Director of the CDC for deposit in the Reserve Fund" (Infectious Diseases Rapid Response Reserve Fund, 42 U.S. Code §247d-4a, 2018).

The Committee's recommended solution is to appropriate funds to the PHEF to be controlled by the secretary of HHS and used subsequent to a declared PHE. This would serve to prevent reliance on supplemental appropriations and congressional approval of funds (DeLauro, n.d.). This solution would also place a cabinet-level official responsible to reporting to Congress that criteria for release of funds have been met, similar to the Stafford Act.[64] Importantly, these funds would "supplement, but do not supplant, other federal, state, and local funds provided for public health grants, awards, contracts, and investigations" (ASPR, 2019) upon declaration of a public health emergency. In an effort to replenish the Public Health Emergency Fund, the Public Health Emergency Response and Accountability Act was introduced in July 2021.[65] The bill also exempts the Public Health Emergency Fund from sequestration, which is a process of automatic, usually across-the-board spending reductions under which budgetary resources are permanently canceled to enforce specific budget policy goals (H.R.5723—116th Congress [2019–2020]: Public health emergency fund act, 2020).

This solution offers several advantages. It utilizes established legislative authority without the need for an additional fund or the need for additional wholly new legislative authority. Adding another new fund may prove confusing to the Congress and difficult for HHS and Office of Management and Budget (OMB) to determine the appropriate target for funds and use for a response. The solution also establishes a ready reserve of funds in the PHEF without fiscal year limitation, thus would not require additional congressional action during an immediate response. Because the fund provides "no-year money that can be carried over if it is not needed right away, it obviates the need for future emergency supplementals" (Alton and Carlin, 2020). Immediately upon declaration of a PHE, it would allow the DGMQ among other HHS operational divisions and their sub-elements to access those funds for testing equipment, other materials, facilities, contract staff support, and quarantine facilities. Moreover, a surge capability could be added to existing legislated authorities that would allow a limited use of these funds prior to a full PHE declaration, much like FEMA's Disaster Relief Fund that can be used prior to a hurricane land fall. The Post-Katrina Emergency Response Act (PKEMRA) could be used as model.[66] This could

---

[64] The Robert T. Stafford Disaster Relief and Emergency Assistance Act, PL 100-707, was signed into law November 23, 1988, and amended the Disaster Relief Act of 1974, PL 93-288. The Stafford Act constitutes the statutory authority for most federal disaster response activities, especially as they pertain to FEMA and FEMA programs.

[65] https://www.congress.gov/bill/117th-congress/senate-bill/2467/text?r=53&s=1 (accessed March 4, 2022).

[66] More information about the Post-Katrina Emergency Response Act is available from https://emilms.fema.gov/is_0822/groups/20.html (accessed March 4, 2022).

be of particular importance for the DGMQ, because border measures must be used very early in an outbreak if they are to have any value in mitigating the spread. The Fund[67] may also be used to facilitate cross-sectorial coordination (Alton and Carlin, 2020). Furthermore, this solution would likely garner public support. A 2016 survey by the Annenberg Public Policy Center shows that 63 percent of people said they support having a fund that the president can draw on to deal with an epidemic without having to ask Congress (Annenberg Public Policy Center, 2016; Kodjak, 2016).

This recommended solution does have potential drawbacks, however. It might easily be ignored by appropriators until a need actually exists, although this might be mitigated by a mandatory appropriation to start to replenish funds as they are used. Additionally, it could detract from congressional appropriation of additional supplemental funds, if the balance is determined at the outset of the response to be sufficient. Congress might also insist on depletion of funds prior to supplemental appropriation. Another disadvantage is its potential to limit the discretion of Congress to further specifically direct appropriations to the fund according to congressional-response priorities, rather than the executive-branch response priorities—although this might be an advantage from the perspective of the executive branch. Importantly, this solution would require the establishment of guard rails and clear congressional reporting. Furthermore, the PHEF does not have a strong existing track record to draw on. HHS officials reported that the Public Health Emergency Fund was last used in 1993, in response to a Hantavirus outbreak in the Southwest United States (GAO, 2018). Since its inception, Congress has only allocated funds to the PHEF on two occasions, first in 1987 and the most recent allocation being in FY1999 (DeLauro, n.d.; NACCHO, 2017). Due to congressional reticence to appropriate to the PHEF, it now sits nearly empty (DeLauro, n.d.). The availability of a standing contingency fund for public health emergencies through legislative reform could be key for a rapid and effective response to infectious disease threats. This notion is further discussed in the "Changes in the DGMQ's Organizational Capacity and Infrastructure" chapter, which details the current DGMQ budget and spending in addition to the emphasis on the urgent need for a sustainable and proactive emergency funding system.

Possible Fund Allocation Criteria and Response/Reporting Requirements

The Committee identified a set of possible criteria for fund allocation:

- When a public health emergency declaration has been made;
- When state or Indian Tribal Government resources are over-

---

[67] 42 U.S. Code §247d—Public health emergencies.

whelmed, similar to requests for support made through FEMA regional offices.[68] Such requests might require (1) confirmation that appropriate action has been taken by local emergency response authorities, (2) a description of efforts and resources utilized to alleviate the emergency, and (3) a description of the type and extent of additional federal assistance required;
- When positivity rates reach an established threshold, which would require the development of escalation criteria based on Laboratory Response Network detection[69] (Katz et al., 2017);
- When the number of refugee arrivals exceeds initial planning figures (CERF, 2017);
- When evidence of a new outbreak at a large scale requires international assistance (CERF, 2017).

The committee also identified a set of reporting and accountability requirements. In addition to normal Public Health Emergency reporting requirements the secretary of HHS must report to Congress: (1) an explanation of why currently nonemergency appropriated funds are insufficient for the response; (2) a description of the activities that will be funded; (3) a preliminary estimate of the amount of funding that will be required for the response; and (4) a description of the STLT or Indian tribal government resources that will also be used to mitigate the public health emergency.

The purpose of specifying criteria and requiring reporting and accountability mechanisms is to ensure that HHS, and its subsidiary the CDC, uses surge funding in an appropriate and effective way, and does not simply use emergency funding for day-to-day operations.

CONCLUSIONS AND RECOMMENDATIONS

Conclusions

By constitutional design, the United States has several levels of government, including federal, state, tribal, territorial, and local. Executive and legislative branches at each level of federal, state, territorial, and tribal governments hold overlapping powers to prevent and manage communicable disease outbreaks, epidemics, and pandemics.

---

[68] More information about FEMA's role in this regard is available from https://www.fema.gov/disaster/how-declared (accessed March 4, 2022).

[69] The Laboratory Response Network is " . . . an integrated network of state and local public health, federal, and military laboratories [that]provides diagnostic capacity to detect biological events and other PHEs across the United States. These networks allow rapid detection and reporting of events at the state and federal levels for decision-making" (Katz et al., 2017).

Conclusion 6-1: While tribes, states, and localities hold primary public health powers, the federal government has an important role to play where purely state or local action cannot avert the risk to the American public. At each level of government there are checks and balances between the legislative, executive, and judicial branches of government. The Constitution creates the judiciary as a third branch of government, charged with interpreting laws and regulations, and ensuring their constitutionality. During the COVID-19 pandemic, some judicial rulings appeared to go beyond settled precedents, thus perhaps unnecessarily delaying or blocking needed public health powers. This constitutional structure entails benefits and disadvantages. When one branch or level of government abdicates its role, redundant responsibilities allow others to step in. Under ideal conditions, shared responsibility empowers governments to cooperate with each level and branch of government playing to its strengths. However, tensions can arise among levels, and even branches, of government. Key actors may fail to act or even block effective science-based measures, sometimes due to politicized or ideologically driven motivations. Even the judiciary has, at times, delayed or blocked urgent public health responses. These factors may undermine a nationally coordinated response. Uncertainty created by recent court rulings could chill agency action if Congress or the executive does not intervene.

Recommendations

Recommendation 6-1: Congress should improve the legal authority and flexibility of the Centers for Disease Control and Prevention (CDC) in responding to public health threats by modernizing and improving the 1944 Public Health Service Act in several ways:
1. Give the CDC authority to effectively act to prevent or mitigate current and future public health threats. The CDC should have the authority it needs but must act consistently with scientific evidence, and only where necessary to prevent the interstate, intrastate, or international spread of infectious diseases. The CDC should also use the least restrictive alternative means that reasonably can be predicted to achieve an important public health objective.
2. Specifically delegate congressional power to reflect what the CDC needs to carry out its mission through evidence-based measures. These delegations should provide the CDC with robust authority and the necessary flexibility to implement science-based public health measures

3. Include protections for individual rights and freedoms including procedural due process, where constitutionally warranted and feasible, to challenge any order under the Act.
4. Ensure that CDC authorities are fairly and equitably utilized.

REFERENCES

Alton, J. B., and E. P. Carlin. 2020. *Now is the time to resource the Public Health Emergency Fund*. https://thehill.com/blogs/congress-blog/healthcare/485163-now-is-the-time-to-resource-the-public-health-emergency-fund (accessed May 22, 2022).

Annenberg Public Policy Center. 2016. *Majority agree on idea of a presidential public health emergency fund*. https://www.annenbergpublicpolicycenter.org/majority-agree-with-the-idea-of-a-presidential-public-health-emergency-fund (accessed May 24, 2022).

ASPR (HHS Office of the Assistant Secretary for Preparedness and Response). 2019. *Public health emergency declaration*. U.S. Department of HHS Office of the Assistant Secretary for Preparedness and Response. https://www.phe.gov/Preparedness/legal/Pages/phedeclaration.aspx (accessed May 22, 2022).

Associated Press. 2020. *Feds drop plan to put quarantined cruise ship passengers in Costa Mesa. KTLA*. https://ktla.com/news/local-news/feds-drop-plan-to-put-quarantined-cruise-ship-passengers-in-costa-mesa (accessed May 22, 2022).

Bajema, K. L., A. M. Oster, O. L. McGovern, S. Lindstrom, M. R. Stenger, T. C. Anderson, C. Isenhour, K. R. Clarke, M. E. Evans, V. T. Chu, H. M. Biggs, H. L. Kirking, S. I. Gerber, A. J. Hall, A. M. Fry, and S. E. Oliver. 2020. Persons evaluated for 2019 novel coronavirus—United States, January 2020. *MMWR: Morbidity and Mortalitly Weekly Report* 69(6):166-170. http://dx.doi.org/10.15585/mmwr.mm6906e1.

Boddie, C. 2015. Federal funding in support of Ebola medical countermeasures R&D. *Health Security* 13(1):3-8. https://doi.org/10.1089/hs.2015.0001.

Brown, C. M., A. E. Aranas, G. A. Benenson, G. Brunette, M. Cetron, T. H. Chen, N. J. Cohen, P. Diaz, Y. Haber, C. R. Hale, K. Holton, K. Kohl, A. W. Le, G. J. Palumbo, K. Pearson, C. R. Phares, F. Alvarado-Ramy, S. Roohi, L. D. Rotz, J. Tappero, F. M. Washburn, J. Watkins, and N. Pesik. 2014. Airport exit and entry screening for Ebola—August–November 10, 2014. *MMWR: Morbidity and Mortalitly Weekly Report* 63(49):1163-1167.

Burel, G. 2020. PPE shortages & funding gaps for pandemics. *Domestic Preparedness* 16(3):6-9.

Canales, K. 2020, February 28. A Southern California city is barring people who were on the coronavirus-stricken *Diamond Princess* cruise ship from entering its town. *Business Insider*. https://www.businessinsider.in/slideshows/miscellaneous/a-southern-california-city-is-banning-people-who-were-on-the-coronavirus-stricken-diamond-princess-cruise-ship-from-entering-their-town/slidelist/74348175.cms (accessed May 22, 2022).

CDC (Centers for Disease Control and Prevention). 2020a. *CDC issues federal quarantine order to repatriated U.S. citizens at March Air Reserve Base*.

CDC. 2020b. *Transcript for CDC media telebriefing: Update on 2019 novel coronavirus (2019-ncov)*. https://www.cdc.gov/media/releases/2020/t0131-2019-novel-coronavirus.html (accessed May 22, 2022).

CDC. 2021a. *CDC issues eviction moratorium order in areas of substantial and high transmission*. https://www.cdc.gov/media/releases/2021/s0803-cdc-eviction-order.html#:~:text=This%20order%20will%20expire%20on,to%20further%20increase%20vaccination%20rates (accessed May 22, 2022).

CDC. 2021b. *Division of Global Migration and Quarantine laws and regulations*. Division of Global Migration and Quarantine. https://www.cdc.gov/ncezid/dgmq/laws-and-regulations.html (accessed May 22, 2022).

CDC. 2021c. *Legal authorities for isolation and quarantine*. https://www.cdc.gov/quarantine/aboutlawsregulationsquarantineisolation.html (accessed March 2, 2022).

CDC. 2022a. *CDC COVID-19 orders for cruise ships*. https://www.cdc.gov/quarantine/cruise/COVID19-cruiseships.html (accessed March 15, 2022).

CDC. 2022b. *Operations manual for CDC's COVID-19 program for cruise ships operating in U.S. waters*. https://www.cdc.gov/quarantine/cruise/COVID19-operations-manual-cso.html (accessed May 22, 2022).

CDC. 2022c. *Requirement for proof of negative COVID-19 test or documentation of recovery from COVID-19*. https://www.cdc.gov/coronavirus/2019-ncov/travelers/testing-international-air-travelers.html#:~:text=Yes%2C%20at%20this%20time%20all,documentation%20of%20recovery%20unless%20exempted (accessed May 22, 2022).

CERF (Central Emergency Response Fund). 2017. *CERF rapid response: Overview of methodology*. https://cerf.un.org/sites/default/files/resources/cerf_ag_rapid_response_en.pdf (accessed May 22, 2022).

Congressional Research Service. 2009. *The 2009 influenza pandemic: An overview*. https://crsreports.congress.gov/product/pdf/R/R40554 (accessed May 22, 2022).

Congressional Research Service. 2021a. *Federal eviction moratoriums in response to the COVID-19 pandemic*.

Congressional Research Service. 2021b. *Scope of CDC authority under Section 361 of the Public Health Service Act (PHSA)*. https://crsreports.congress.gov/product/pdf/R/R46758 (accessed May 22, 2022).

DeBonis, M. 2021. After Kentucky devastation, critics seize on Rand Paul's record opposing disaster bills. *The Washington Post*, December 14.

DeLauro, R. n.d.. *Why we need a public health emergency fund*. https://delauro.house.gov/public-health-emergency-fund (accessed March 20, 2022).

FEMA (Federal Emergency Management Agency). 2013. *Disaster relief fund: Appropriation overview*. https://www.fema.gov/pdf/about/budget/11f_fema_disaster_relief_fund_dhs_fy13_cj.pdf (accessed May 20, 2022).

GAO (General Accounting Office). 2018. *Opioid crisis: Status of public health emergency authorities*. https://www.gao.gov/products/gao-18-685r (accessed May 15, 2022).

Gostin, L. O. 2018. Public health emergency preparedness: Globalizing risk, localizing threats. *JAMA* 320(17):1743-1744.

Gostin, L. O. 2021. *Global health security: A blueprint for the future*. Cambridge, MA: Harvard University Press.

Gostin, L. O., and J. G. Hodge. 2017. Reforming federal public health powers. *JAMA* 317(12):1211.

Gostin, L. O., and D. Hosie. 2022. No matter how you feel about masks, you should be alarmed by this judge's decision. *The New York Times*, April 25.

Gostin, L. O., W. E. Parmet, and S. Rosenbaum. 2022. The U.S. Supreme Court's rulings on large business and health care worker vaccine mandates. *JAMA* 327(8):713.

H.R.5723—116th Congress (2019–2020): *Public Health Emergency Fund Act*. (2020). https://www.congress.gov/bill/116th-congress/house-bill/5723 (accessed May 24, 2022).

Katz, R., A. Attal-Juncqua, and J. E. Fischer. 2017. Funding public health emergency preparedness in the United States. *American Journal of Public Health* 107(S2):S148-S152.

Kodjak, A. 2016. *A permanent fund that could help fight Zika exists, but it's empty*. https://www.npr.org/sections/health-shots/2016/06/03/480565668/a-permanent-fund-to-help-fight-zika-exists-but-its-empty (accessed March 20, 2022).

Montoya-Galvez, C. 2022. Biden administration defends Trump-era migrant expulsions citing "serious" COVID-19 risk. https://www.cbsnews.com/news/immigration-title-42-biden-trump-migrant-expulsions (accessed February 28, 2022).

Mortenson, J. D., and N. Bagley. 2021. Delegation at the founding. *Columbia Law Review* 121(2):277-368. https://repository.law.umich.edu/articles/2200.

NACCHO (National Association of County and City Health Officials). 2017. Statement of policy: Public health emergency response fund. https://www.naccho.org/uploads/downloadable-resources/17-05-Public-Health-Emergency-Response-Fund.pdf (accessed March 15, 2022).

O'Toole, T. 2007. Testimony given to the U.S. Congress, Senate, Committee on Homeland Security and Governmental Affairs. In *Six years after anthrax: Are we better prepared to respond to bioterrorism?* United States Senate Committee on Homeland Security and Governmental Affairs.

Parmet, W. E. 2007. Legal power and legal rights—isolation and quarantine in the case of drug-resistant tuberculosis. *New England Journal of Medicine* 357(5):433-435.

Pereira, I. 2020. Feds backtrack on transfer of quarantined coronavirus patients to Alabama. *ABC News*. https://abcnews.go.com/Health/feds-backtrack-transfer-quarantined-coronavirus-patients-alabama/story?id=69162771 (accessed May 24, 2022).

Simon, S., and M. Evstatieva. 2020. A revamped Strategic National Stockpile still can't match the pandemic's latest surge [interview]. November 23. https://www.npr.org/transcripts/937978556 (accessed May 24, 2022).

U.S. Embassy & Consulates in the United Kingdom. 2021. *Important information about COVID-19 tests for travelers to and from the UK and U.S.* https://uk.usembassy.gov/information-about-COVID-tests-for-travelers-from-the-uk-to-us (accessed March 20, 2022).

Whitcomb, D. 2020. Trump administration backs off sending coronavirus patients to Alabama governor. *Reuters*. https://www.reuters.com/article/us-china-health-usa-alabama/trump-administration-backs-off-sending-coronavirus-patients-to-alabama-governor-idUSKCN20I01W (accessed May 24, 2022).

Appendix A

Biographical Sketches of Committee Members and Staff

COMMITTEE MEMBERS

Georges C. Benjamin, M.D., (**Committee Chair**) is a well-known health policy leader, practitioner, and administrator. He currently serves as the executive director of the American Public Health Association (APHA), the nation's oldest and largest organization of public health professionals. He is also a former secretary of health for the state of Maryland. Dr. Benjamin is a graduate of the Illinois Institute of Technology and the University of Illinois College of Medicine. He is board certified in internal medicine, a master of the American College of Physicians, a fellow of the National Academy of Public Administration, a fellow emeritus of the American College of Emergency Physicians, and a member of the National Academy of Medicine. At APHA he serves as the publisher for the American Journal of Public Health, The Nation's Health newspaper, and APHA Press, the association's book company. He serves on several nonprofit boards, such as Research!America, the Truth Foundation, the Environmental Defense Fund, Ceres, and the Reagan-Udall Foundation. He is also a former member of the National Infrastructure Advisory Council, a council that advises the president on how to best assure the security of the nation's critical infrastructure.

Ana Abraído-Lanza, Ph.D., is vice dean of the School of Global Public Health and professor in the Department of Social and Behavioral Sciences at New York University (NYU). Prior to joining NYU, she was professor of sociomedical sciences at the Mailman School of Public Health of Columbia University. She received her Ph.D. in psychology from The Graduate School at the City University of New York. Her research expertise includes the cultural, psychological, social, and structural factors that affect health, psychological well-being, mortality among Latinos, and the health of immigrant Latinos. She has served as a committee or board member on the Hispanic-Serving Health Professions Schools, the Community Task Force on Preventive Services of the Centers for Disease Control and Prevention (from 2006–2011), and several National Institutes of Health review groups among others. Dr. Abraído-Lanza's honors and awards include being selected as a Columbia University Provost Leadership Fellow, as well as receiving the Teaching Excellence Award from the Mailman School of Public Health of Columbia University, a Dalmas A. Taylor Distinguished Contributions Award from the Minority Fellowship Program of the American Psychological Association, and the Student Assembly Public Health Mentoring Award from the American Public Health Association.

Michele Barry, M.D., FACP, FASTMH, is the Drs. Ben and A. Jess Shenson Professor of Medicine and Tropical Diseases at Stanford University, where she is the director of the Center for Innovation in Global Health and senior associate dean for Global Health. She is past president of the American Society of Tropical Medicine and Hygiene (ASTMH), where she led an educational initiative in tropical medicine and travelers' health, which culminated in diploma courses in tropical medicine both in the United States and overseas, as well as a U.S. certification exam. Dr. Barry is an elected member of the National Academy of Medicine and an elected member of The American Academy of Arts and Sciences. She has been selected for Best Doctors in America and currently sits on the National Academies' Board on Global Health. She is chair of the board of directors for the Consortium of Universities for Global Health and is a recipient of the Ben Kean Medal given every 3 years by the ASTMH to the outstanding tropical disease educator in the United States. She is a recipient of the Elizabeth Blackwell Award for mentoring women in the United States toward careers in medicine, and is the founder of the Gates-funded WomenLift program, a global women's leadership program in the private and public health sectors. She has written on the impact of COVID-19 on female academics, among other areas in tropical diseases, and global and refugee health.

Ietza Bojorquez, M.D., MSc, Ph.D., is a professor-researcher at the Department of Population Studies, El Colegio de la Frontera Norte. From 2007–2010 she was the director of research at Mexico's Directorate of Epidemiology, Ministry of Health, where she was in charge of the surveillance system for the H1N1 pandemic of 2009. She conducts research from a social epidemiology/social determinants of health perspective. Her research focuses on mental health, migrant health, and the inclusion of migrants in health policies. Since 2018, she has been responsible for the Surveys on Migration in Mexico's Borders, an interinstitutional effort to track migration flows in Northern and Southern Mexico. Her recent research projects address the health of Mexican migrants in the Mexico–U.S. migration corridor, as well as non-Mexican in-transit migrants and asylum seekers in Mexico. She has been part of research teams studying the "migrant caravans" in the Mexico–U.S. border. She is working on a project on the health-related impact of the COVID-19 pandemic on migrants in Mexico, which is funded by Mexico's Ministry of Health through an agreement with the U.S. Centers for Disease Control and Prevention. She is a member of the board of the Latin America node, Lancet Commission on Migration and Health. She provided uncompensated expert public health evidence for the American Civil Liberties Union (ACLU) for litigation against the detention of migrants during the COVID-19 pandemic, which has been resolved, and has signed an ACLU declaration opposing the use of Title 42 to return asylum seekers at the U.S. border. She is part of Mexico's National System of Researchers. She holds an M.D., an MSc in Public Health, and a Ph.D. in Epidemiology.

J. Bradley Dickerson, Ph.D., leads the Global Chemical and Biological Security (GCBS) group at Sandia National Laboratories (SNL). The GCBS group also works with the Centers for Disease Control and Prevention's (CDC's) Center for Surveillance, Epidemiology, and Laboratory Services on laboratory biorisk management through an interagency agreement between the CDC and SNL. Dr. Dickerson has held numerous leadership positions within the U.S. government. Prior to joining SNL, he served as the principal scientific officer in the Department of Justice's National Security Division, working for the Committee on Foreign Investment in the United States. Prior to that, Dr. Dickerson served as the senior biodefense advisor and the director of chemical security policy at the Department of Homeland Security (DHS). At DHS he was responsible for the development and implementation of policies associated with chemical and biological defense, pandemic preparedness, and infectious disease–related border and transportation issues. Dr. Dickerson also led the policy and strategy component of the Office of Public Health Preparedness and Response at the CDC. He worked in the U.S. Senate as Senator Bob Corker's foreign relations legislative assistant. Prior to government service, Dr. Dickerson was a researcher at St. Jude Children's Research Hospital and a pharmaceutical chemist at Schering-Plough Health Care Products. Dr. Dickerson holds degrees in chemistry (B.S.), biomedical engineering (M.S.), and biochemistry (Ph.D.). He is a member of the Council on Foreign Relations.

Lawrence Gostin is University Professor, Georgetown University's highest academic rank, and founding O'Neill Chair in Global Health Law. He directs the World Health Organization Center on National and Global Health Law. Professor Gostin served on two global commissions on the Ebola epidemic, and was senior advisor to the United Nations secretary general's post-Ebola Commission. He served on the drafting committee for the G-7 Summit on global health security. A member of the National Academy of Medicine, he also serves on the National Academies' Global Health Board. The National Academy and American Public Health Association awarded him their Distinguished Achievement Award. He's a fellow of the Royal Society of Public Health and faculty of public health (UK). President Obama appointed Gostin to the President's National Cancer Advisory Board. The National Consumer Council (UK) bestowed the Rosemary Delbridge Memorial Award for the person "who has most influenced Parliament and government to act for the welfare of society."

Moon Kim, M.D., M.P.H., is a medical epidemiologist in charge of the Hospital Outbreak and Biothreat Response Unit of the Los Angeles County Department of Public Health's (CDPH) Acute Communicable Disease Control (ACDC) Program and is responsible for investigating hospital outbreaks, emerging diseases (e.g., viral hemorrhagic fevers), and suspected cases of bioterrorism including anthrax, botulism, and smallpox. She has over 19 years of experience leading a variety of public health investigations and outbreaks (e.g., fungal endophthalmitis, hepatitis A, non-tuberculous mycobacteria, Legionellosis, aspergillosis, medical-device and product contamination) and has worked with the Centers for Disease Control and Prevention (CDC) and CDPH investigating numerous outbreaks including those that are multijurisdictional.

During the COVID-19 pandemic, Dr. Kim served as the public health liaison to the Los Angeles CDC Quarantine Station, which included traveler monitoring and screening activities, following up on Do Not Board orders, overseeing outbreaks in the transportation sector (e.g., airlines, metro, transit), and planning/responding to maritime issues with the CDC. During the Ebola 2014–2016 outbreak in West Africa, she oversaw Ebola planning and response activities for suspected cases and traveler monitoring/screening activities for ACDC. She is board certified in infectious diseases and also received her masters of public health from the UCLA School of Public Health.

Lonnie King, Ph.D., is the Academy Professor and Dean Emeritus at The Ohio State University College of Veterinary Medicine. He previously was dean of the College of Veterinary Medicine at Ohio State, dean of the College of Veterinary Medicine at Michigan State University, and interim dean and university vice-president for agriculture at the College of Food, Agriculture and Environmental Sciences at Ohio State. Dr. King served as the director of the National Center of Zoonotic, Vector-Borne, and Enteric Diseases with the Centers for Disease Control and Prevention (CDC) from 2006–2009, and was the administrator for the Animal and Plant Health Inspection Service at the U.S. Department of Agriculture, where he also served as the deputy administrator for veterinary services and the chief veterinary officer for the United States. His expertise focuses on emerging infectious diseases and zoonoses, food safety, global health, public health, and One Health. Dr. King has been active in antimicrobial resistance issues and has worked at the interface of human and animal diseases. He is a member of the American Veterinary Medical Association and is a member of the National Academy of Medicine, where he served as vice chair of the Forum on Microbial Threats for almost 10 years. He has been honored with global awards in One Health, and Meritorious Service via the World Organization for Animal Health. He currently is serving for a sixth year as co-chair for the PACCARB (President's Advisory Council to Combat Antibiotic Resistant Bacteria).

Marcelle Layton, M.D., is the assistant commissioner for the Bureau of Communicable Disease at the New York City (NYC) Department of Health and Mental Hygiene. As of December 1, 2021, she is the chief medical officer for the Council of State and Territorial Epidemiologists (CSTE). Dr. Layton has participated as a member of the National Academies' Forum on Microbial Threats; the University of Pittsburgh's Center for Civilian Biosecurity; the Executive Session on Domestic Preparedness of the John F. Kennedy School of Government, Harvard University; the IOM Committee on Effectiveness of National Biosurveillance Systems: Biowatch and the Public Health System; the H1N1 Subcommittee to the President's Council of Advisors on Science and Technology; the Centers for Disease Control and Prevention's Board of Scientific Counselors (from 2008 to 2011); and the National Institutes of Health's National Science Advisory Board for Biosecurity. She was previously on the Executive Board of the CSTE from 2013 to 2020.

Dr. Layton played a key role in NYC's public health response to the appearance of West Nile virus in 1999 and the attacks on the World Trade Center and intentional anthrax release in 2001, and has led the surveillance response to multiple emergencies in recent years including the 2009 H1N1 pandemic, the threat of imported Ebola and Zika virus, and the current COVID-19 pandemic.

Stephen Ostroff, Ph.D., served as the deputy commissioner for foods and veterinary medicine at the U.S. Food and Drug Administration (FDA) until early 2019. In addition to that position, he also served as the FDA's chief scientist and acting commissioner on two occasions. Before joining the FDA, Dr. Ostroff worked at the Centers for Disease Control and Prevention (CDC) from 1986–2005, serving as deputy director of the National Center for Infectious Diseases (NCID) and NCID associate director for epidemiologic science. He attained the rank of Assistant Surgeon General in the U.S. Public Health Service Commissioned Corps. Between leaving the CDC and joining the FDA, Dr. Ostroff led the Bureau of Epidemiology and served as acting physician general at the Pennsylvania Department of Health in Harrisburg.

Dr. Ostroff served as a member of the Healthy to Sail panel, which advised the Royal Caribbean and Norwegian cruise lines on the development and implementation of COVID-19 health and safety protocols between June 2020 and April 2021. He continued to serve as a compensated consultant to Norwegian through October 2021, including providing declaratory statements in July–August 2021 in litigation between Norwegian cruise lines and the State of Florida regarding the importance of verifying COVID-19 vaccination status.

He is a medical editor of the CDC's Health Information for International Travel (the Yellow Book). Dr. Ostroff received his medical degree from the University of Pennsylvania School of Medicine and did residency training in internal medicine at the University of Colorado Health Sciences Center and in preventive medicine at the CDC. He holds adjunct faculty appointments at the Penn State College of Medicine and the University of Pittsburgh Graduate School of Public Health.

Edward T. Ryan, M.D., is a physician, scientist, educator, and public health advocate. Dr. Ryan received his undergraduate degree from Princeton University and his doctorate in medicine from Harvard University. He performed his graduate medical training at Massachusetts General Hospital in Boston. Dr. Ryan is a professor of immunology and infectious diseases at the Harvard T. H. Chan School of Public Health, professor of medicine at Harvard Medical School, and director of global infectious diseases at Massachusetts General Hospital. Dr. Ryan's efforts focus on mitigating the burden and impact of global infectious diseases. Dr. Ryan is a National Institutes of Health (NIH) MERIT Awardee. Dr. Ryan's scholarly efforts include over 240 peer-reviewed publications, and 90 editorials, chapters, and reviews. He also serves in a number of editorial capacities and has served on expert and advisory committees and working groups for the World Health Organization (WHO), the Institute of Medicine/National Academy of Sciences, the Centers for Disease Control and Prevention, the NIH, the Wellcome Trust, and PATH (formerly the Program for Appropriate Technologies in Health). Dr. Ryan is a previous president of the American Society of Tropical Medicine & Hygiene (ASTMH), and is a fellow of the

American College of Physicians, the Infectious Diseases Society of America, the ASTMH, and the American Academy of Microbiology.

Alessandro Vespignani is the director of the Network Science Institute and Sternberg Family Distinguished University Professor with interdisciplinary appointments in the College of Computer and Information Science, College of Science, and the Bouvé College of Health Sciences at Northeastern University. Before joining Northeastern University, Mr. Vespignani was J. H. Rudy Professor of Informatics and Computing at Indiana University, serving as the director of the Center for Complex Networks and Systems Research and the associate director of the Pervasive Technology Institute. His research interests include complex systems and networks, and the data-driven computational modeling of epidemics. Mr. Vespignani's recent work has focused on modeling the spatial spread of epidemics, including the realistic and data-driven modeling of emerging infectious diseases. He is a fellow of the American Physical Society and the Network Science Society. He has been inducted into the Academia Europaea (section Physics and Engineering), and received the Doctorate Honoris Causa from Delft University of Technology in the Netherlands and the John Graunt award for extraordinary achievements in one of the population sciences.

C. Jason Wang, M.D., Ph.D., is director of the Center for Policy, Outcomes, and Prevention and co-chair of the mobile health group in the Center for Population Health Sciences at Stanford University. He is a professor of pediatrics and health policy at Stanford University. He received his B.S. from MIT, M.D. from Harvard Medical School, and Ph.D. in policy analysis from RAND. After pediatric residency training at the University of California, San Francisco, he worked in Greater China with McKinsey and Company. In 2000, he served as the project manager for Taiwan's Healthcare Reform Taskforce. He is currently on the RAND Health Board. Dr. Wang has conducted an independent evaluation on Taiwan's COVID-19 response and has published extensively on both Taiwan's experience as well as other ways to improve the detection, containment, and mitigation of COVID-19.

Among his honors, he was selected as the student speaker for the Harvard Medical School commencement ceremony in 1996, is a recipient of the 2011 National Institutes of Health Director's New Innovator Award, and was an invited speaker for the Johns Hopkins Bloomberg School of Public Health's 100th Year, Child Health Policy Symposium.

Rueben Warren, Ph.D., M.P.H., DrPh, is professor of bioethics and director of the National Center for Bioethics in Research and Health Care at Tuskegee University. He has served as dean of the School of Dentistry at Meharry Medical College (MMC) (1983–1988); associate director for minority health at the Centers for Disease Control and Prevention (1988–1997); associate director for urban affairs at the Agency for Toxic Substances and Disease Registry (1997–2004); and director of infrastructure development at the National Institute for Minority Health and Health Disparities (part-time, 2004–2007). His professional and research interests include health services research, minority health, public health, ethics and theology, environmental justice, and international health. In 1999, Dr. Warren received the Distinguished Harvard Alumni Award. From MMC he has received an honorary degree of Doctor of Medical Science (1999), the President's Distinguished Service Award (2001), a School of Dentistry Dean Emeritus (2003) appointment, and an honorary Doctor of Humane Letters (2013). From the NYU School of Dentistry, he received the Michael C. Alfano Award for Promoting Diversity (2010). He earned a BA in biology at San Francisco State University; a doctor of dental surgery at MMC; an MPH, DrPH, and teaching fellowship at Harvard School of Public Health; residency in dental public health at the Harvard School of Dental Medicine (board certified in dental public health); a masters of divinity at the Interdenominational Theological Center; and a certificate in bioethics at Georgetown University.

STAFF

Liz Ashby is an associate program officer with the Board on Global Health, where she supports the Forum on Microbial Threats. Her previous work with the National Academies includes writing, research, and program support for the studies Globally Resilient Supply Chains for Pandemic and Seasonal Influenza Vaccines and Vaccine Research and Development to Advance Pandemic and Seasonal Influenza Preparedness and Response: Lessons from COVID-19. Previously, she conducted research in collaboration with the PREDICT project for global disease surveillance to assess risk factors for zoonotic disease transmission in Kenya. She also worked with a private consulting company to apply social marketing interventions and innovative technologies to pressing global health issues. Her primary interests include applying a One Health lens to analyze challenges related to emerging pandemic threats. She has an M.S. in environmental science from George Mason University, where she studied the intersection of human, animal, and environmental health.

Elizabeth Ferré, M.P.H., is a research associate with the Board on Global Health in the Health and Medicine Division at the National Academies of Sciences, Engineering, and Medicine in Washington, DC. She is currently working on the Analysis to Enhance the Effectiveness of the Federal Quarantine Station Network Based on Lessons from the COVID-19 Pandemic project. Previously, she has worked on sustainable financing methods for global health security and preparedness for the Global Health Security Agenda Consortium through Gryphon Scientific. Her interests lie in anticipation, prevention, detection, and response to infectious diseases, global health security, pandemic preparedness, and achievement of health equity. She is originally from Boston, Massachusetts, and attended James Madison University for a bachelor's of science in public health and then completed a master's of public health with a concentration in global health from the University of Maryland School of Medicine.

Rose Marie Martinez, Sc.D., has been the Director of the Health and Medicine Division's (formerly the Institute of Medicine's) Board on Population Health and Public Health Practice since 1999. Prior to joining the Academies, Dr. Martinez was a senior health researcher at Mathematica Policy Research (1995–1999) where she conducted research on the impact of health system change on the public health infrastructure, access to care for vulnerable populations, managed care, and the health care workforce. She is a former assistant director for health financing and policy with the U.S. General Accounting Office and served for 6 years directing research studies for the Regional Health Ministry of Madrid, Spain.

Julie A. Pavlin, M.D., Ph.D., M.P.H., is the director of the Board on Global Health and is board certified in preventive medicine and public health. She is a retired Colonel in the U.S. Army with previous assignments including the Armed Forces Research Institute of Medical Sciences in Bangkok, Thailand; the Walter Reed Army Institute of Research; and the U.S. Army Medical Research Institute for Infectious Diseases. After she retired from active duty, she served as the deputy director at the Armed Forces Health Surveillance Center. She concentrated most of her time with the Department of Defense in the design of real-time disease surveillance systems and was a cofounder of the International Society for Disease Surveillance.

Emilie Ryan-Castillo is a research assistant with the Board on Global Health. She has a B.S. in public health from American University. In the past, she was a program assistant at FHI 360 and worked on diabetes prevention and childhood obesity research projects. In this role, she helped execute several large meetings bringing together the top researchers from the Centers for Disease Control and Prevention, the National Institutes of Health, the U.S. Department of Agriculture, and the Robert Wood Johnson Foundation for the National Collaborative on Childhood Obesity Research. She recently served as a rural community health volunteer in Peace Corps Benin, where she worked on improving maternal health, vaccination rates, and community outreach at a local clinic in the Borgou Department.

Tequam Worku, M.P.H., is a program officer for the Board on Global Health at the National Academies of Sciences, Engineering, and Medicine. She previously worked at the Association of State and Territorial Health Officials as a senior analyst for Clinical to Community Connections, managing federally funded projects on community health workers and ending the HIV epidemic. Her past experience also includes working on federally funded projects related to chronic diseases and the development of healthy communities, including the promotion of healthy aging and hypertension prevention and control (the Million Hearts Initiative). Tequam has worked on various research projects on topics including breast cancer disparities and cultural competency in health care. Additionally, she has worked internationally supporting data analysis and knowledge management efforts. She is committed to efforts aimed at bridging disparities in health and has been actively involved in health-equity initiatives. She earned her B.A. in biology from University of Maryland Baltimore County and an M.P.H. from The George Washington University and is currently pursuing a DrPH at Morgan State University.

Appendix B

Agendas: Open Committee Meetings

This appendix presents the agendas for the open portions of the committee's meetings, at which a wide range of experts provided invaluable input to the committee's deliberations.

Committee on the Analysis to Enhance the Effectiveness of the Federal Quarantine Station Network Based on Lessons from the COVID-19 Pandemic

November Meetings
November 8, 15, and 18, 2021
November 8, 2021, 11:00 a.m. to 3 p.m. ET
November 15, 2021, 11:00 a.m. to 2 p.m. ET
November 18, 2021, 1 p.m. to 4 p.m. ET

Meeting Objectives

- Conduct committee and staff introductions
- Orient the committee to the National Academies consensus study process
- Conduct the bias and conflicts of interest discussion
- Hold an open session to hear from sponsoring agencies on their perspectives for the statement of task
- Hear from external speakers to get a landscape of the issues related to each task
- Discuss the statement of task and agree on an approach for completing the study
- Identify information needs and a work plan for addressing the statement of task
- Determine the framework for the report

Monday, November 8, 2021

OPEN SESSION

11:00 a.m.   **Welcome, Introductions, and Meeting's Objective**
GEORGES C. BENJAMIN, *Committee Chair*
Executive Director
American Public Health Association
- Discuss the plan for this meeting, including expectations for where the committee wants to be with regard to the main areas of information by the end of the third day

SPONSOR BRIEFING: DISCUSSION OF THE STATEMENT OF TASK

11:10 a.m.   **Division of Global Migration and Quarantine Overview and COVID-19 Regulatory Activities**
JENNIFER BUIGUT
Associate Director for Policy and Regulatory Affairs
Division of Global Migration and Quarantine
U.S. Centers for Disease Control and Prevention

BRIAN MASKERY
Health Economist
Division of Global Migration and Quarantine
U.S. Centers for Disease Control and Prevention

11:30 a.m.   **Recommendations and Implementation from the 2006 National Academies Report**
MARTIN CETRON
Director
Division of Global Migration and Quarantine
U.S. Centers for Disease Control and Prevention

11:50 a.m.   **Discussion with Committee**

12:00 p.m.   **Break**

End of Open Session

APPENDIX B   *219*

SPEAKER AND DISCUSSION ON HISTORY OF BORDER QUARANTINE

1:15 p.m.   **Welcome and Introduction from the Committee Chair**
            GEORGES C. BENJAMIN, *Committee Chair*
            Executive Director
            American Public Health Association

1:16 p.m.   **Quarantine in the "Bad Old Days": The View from New York Harbor**
            HOWARD MARKEL
            Director, Center for the History of Medicine
            University of Michigan

1:45 p.m.   **Discussion with Committee**

2:15 p.m.   **ADJOURN OPEN SESSION AND DAY 1 OF MEETING**

Monday, November 15, 2021

SESSION IV—CDC BORDER QUARANTINE STATION NETWORK

11:00 a.m. **Welcome and Introduction from the Committee Chair**
            GEORGES C. BENJAMIN, *Committee Chair*
            Executive Director
            American Public Health Association

11:05 a.m. **DHS Support to DGMQ: A Collaborative Approach**
            GARY RASICOT
            Acting Assistant Secretary
            Countering Weapons of Mass Destruction
            U. S. Department of Homeland Security

11:30 a.m. **Q&A**

11:45 a.m. **To Screen or Not to Screen? There's More to Border Health than Interventions at the Border**
            CLIVE M. BROWN
            Chief, Quarantine and Border Health Services
            Division of Global Migration and Quarantine
            U.S. Centers for Disease Control and Prevention

FRANCISCO ALVARADO-RAMY
Chief Medical Officer, Quarantine and Border Health Services
Division of Global Migration and Quarantine
U.S. Centers for Disease Control and Prevention

ANDY KLEVOS
Regional Officer in Charge, Quarantine and Border Health Services
Division of Global Migration and Quarantine
U.S. Centers for Disease Control and Prevention

12:15 p.m.   Q&A

End of Open Session

Thursday, November 18, 2021

OPEN SESSION

REFUGEES AND MIGRATION

1:00 p.m.   **Welcome and Introduction from the Committee Chair**
GEORGES C. BENJAMIN, *Committee Chair*
Executive Director
American Public Health Association

1:05 p.m.   The **CDC's Role in Immigrant, Refugee, and Migrant Health**
NINA MARANO
Chief, Immigrant, Refugee, and Migrant Health Branch
Division of Global Migration and Quarantine
U.S. Centers for Disease Control and Prevention

EMILY JENTES
Lead of Domestic Team, Immigrant, Refugee, and Migrant Health Branch
Division of Global Migration and Quarantine
U.S. Centers for Disease Control and Prevention

APPENDIX B

    EDGAR MONTERROSO
    Senior Epidemiologist, Southwest Border Migrant Health Task Force
    Division of Global Migration and Quarantine
    U.S. Centers for Disease Control and Prevention

    ALFONSO RODRIGUEZ LAINZ
    Epidemiologist, Southwest Border Migrant Health Task Force
    Division of Global Migration and Quarantine
    U.S. Centers for Disease Control and Prevention

1:40 p.m. Discussion with Committee

    End of Open Session

December Meetings

December 6, 7, and 8, 2021
December 6, 2021, 12:00 p.m. to 3 p.m. ET
December 7, 2021, 12:00 p.m. to 3 p.m. ET
December 8, 2021, 1 p.m. to 4 p.m. ET

Meeting Objectives

- Orient the committee to the National Academies consensus study process
- Hold an open session to hear from sponsoring agencies and leadership on their perspectives for the statement of task and the responsibility of the Division of Global Migration and Quarantine
- Understand how the Division of Global Migration and Quarantine evaluates and monitors programs and policy
- Identify information needs and a work plan for addressing the statement of task
- Determine the framework for the report

Monday, December 6, 2021

OPEN SESSION

12:45 p.m. Welcome and Meeting's Objective
    GEORGES C. BENJAMIN, *Committee Chair*
    Executive Director
    American Public Health Association

SESSION II—SPONSOR PERSPECTIVE: DISCUSSION OF THE STATEMENT OF TASK

12:45 p.m. **DGMQ Perspective on Scope of Statement of Task**
JENNIFER BUIGUT
Associate Director for Policy and Regulatory Affairs
Division of Global Migration and Quarantine
U.S. Centers for Disease Control and Prevention

BRIAN MASKERY
Health Economist
Division of Global Migration and Quarantine
U.S. Centers for Disease Control and Prevention

MARTIN CETRON
Director
Division of Global Migration and Quarantine
U.S. Centers for Disease Control and Prevention

SESSION III—PERSPECTIVES FROM CDC LEADERSHIP ON DGMQ NEEDS

1:30 p.m. **Perspective from CDC Leadership**
RIMA KHABBAZ
Director, National Center for Emerging and Zoonotic Infectious Diseases
U.S. Centers for Disease Control and Prevention

JAY BUTLER
Deputy Director for Infectious Disease
U.S. Centers for Disease Control and Prevention

2:00 p.m. **Discussion with Committee**

2:30 p.m. **End of Open Session**

APPENDIX B

Tuesday, December 7, 2021

OPEN SESSION

SESSION V—LOCAL QUARANTINE STATIONS AND PUBLIC HEALTH COLLABORATION

12:00 p.m.	**Welcome and Introduction from the Moderator** LONNIE J. KING Academy Professor and Dean Emeritus College of Veterinary Medicine The Ohio State University
12:05 p.m.	**Quarantine Station Operations and Staffing** FRANCISCO ALVARADO-RAMY Chief Medical Officer, Quarantine and Border Health Services Division of Global Migration and Quarantine U.S. Centers for Disease Control and Prevention TAI-HO CHEN Medical Officer, Quarantine and Border Health Services Division of Global Migration and Quarantine U.S. Centers for Disease Control and Prevention ANDY KLEVOS Regional Officer in Charge, Quarantine and Border Health Services Division of Global Migration and Quarantine U.S. Centers for Disease Control and Prevention ERICA SISON Officer in Charge, CDC Newark Quarantine Station Division of Global Migration and Quarantine U.S. Centers for Disease Control and Prevention CLIVE M. BROWN Chief, Quarantine and Border Health Services Division of Global Migration and Quarantine U.S. Centers for Disease Control and Prevention
12:35 p.m.	**Q&A**

1:05 p.m.   Partnerships with Local Agencies
            Moderated by Moon Kim and Marci Layton
            KATHERINE FELDMAN
            Chief Public Health Scientist
            Maryland Department of Health

            MATTHEW ZAHN
            Medical Director
            Orange County Health Care Agency in California

            DEEPAM THOMAS
            Foodborne/Respiratory Illness Unit Coordinator
            State of New Jersey Department of Health

            CHRISTOPHER SHIELDS
            Assistant Commissioner for Preparedness and Response
            Chicago Department of Public Health

1:35 p.m.   Q&A

2:05 p.m.   Break

SESSION VI—DATA AND EVALUATION

2:10 p.m.   Introduction from the Moderator
            STEPHEN M. OSTROFF
            Adjunct Professor
            University of Pittsburgh Graduate School of Public Health

2:15 p.m.   The Quarantine Activity Reporting System and
            Monitoring/Evaluation
            FRANCISCO ALVARADO-RAMY
            Chief Medical Officer, Quarantine and Border Health
            Services
            Division of Global Migration and Quarantine
            U.S. Centers for Disease Control and Prevention

            TAI-HO CHEN
            Medical Officer, Quarantine and Border Health Services
            Division of Global Migration and Quarantine
            U.S. Centers for Disease Control and Prevention

DAISY CHRISTENSEN
Associate Chief of Science, Quarantine, and Border Health Services
Division of Global Migration and Quarantine
U.S. Centers for Disease Control and Prevention

CLIVE M. BROWN
Chief, Quarantine and Border Health Services
Division of Global Migration and Quarantine
U.S. Centers for Disease Control and Prevention

ARDATH GRILLS
Health Scientist
Division of Global Migration and Quarantine
U.S. Centers for Disease Control and Prevention

3:00 p.m. **ADJOURN**

Wednesday, December 8, 2021

OPEN SESSION

SESSION VII—FURTHER DISCUSSION WITH CDC LEADERSHIP

1:00 p.m.	**Welcome and Introduction from the Committee Chair** GEORGES C. BENJAMIN, *Committee Chair* Executive Director American Public Health Association
1:05 p.m.	**Perspective from CDC Leadership** ANNE SCHUCHAT Former Principal Deputy Director U.S. Centers for Disease Control and Prevention
1:40 p.m.	**Discussion with Committee**
2:00 p.m.	**End of Open Session**

January Meetings

January 19, 20, and 21, 2022
January 19, 2022, 10 a.m. to 1 p.m. ET
January 20, 2022, 2 p.m. to 5 p.m. ET
January 21, 2022, 11 a.m. to 2 p.m. ET

Meeting Objectives

- Hear international perspectives on COVID-19 mitigation measures
- Hear perspectives from the private industry (cruise and airline) and discuss their relationship with CDC
- Discuss legal and regulatory issues pertinent to U.S. quarantine stations
- Identify best practices in response efforts and determine measures that are applicable to the U.S. context at national, state, and local levels
- Begin the development of draft conclusions and recommendations for the report

---

Wednesday, January 19, 2022

OPEN SESSION

SESSION I—INTERNATIONAL PERSPECTIVES

10:00 a.m. Welcome and Meeting's Objective
GEORGES C. BENJAMIN, *Committee Chair*
Executive Director
American Public Health Association

10:05 a.m. International Perspectives on COVID-19 Mitigation
GABRIEL LEUNG
Dean of Medicine
The University of Hong Kong

JONG-KOO LEE
Professor
Seoul National University College of Medicine

C. J. CHEN
Distinguished Professor
Genomics Research Center, Academia Sinica, Taiwan

APPENDIX B 227

     CHORH CHUAN TAN
     Chief Health Scientist, Executive Director
     Office for Healthcare Transformation
     Ministry of Health, Singapore

     ALAIN BOUCARD
     Senior Quarantine Advisor
     Public Health Agency, Canada

     DAVID HEYMANN
     Professor of Infectious Disease Epidemiology
     London School of Hygiene & Tropical Medicine

11:35 a.m. **Q&A**

12:10 p.m. **Break**

     End of Open Session

Thursday, January 20, 2022

OPEN SESSION

SESSION III—INTERNATIONAL AND CRUISE INDUSTRY PERSPECTIVES

2:00 p.m. **Welcome and Introduction from the Moderator**
     GEORGES C. BENJAMIN, *COMMITTEE CHAIR*
     EXECUTIVE DIRECTOR
     AMERICAN PUBLIC HEALTH ASSOCIATION

2:05 p.m. **Perspectives on COVID-19 Mitigation—Australia**
     KARIN LEDER
     Professor, Epidemiology and Preventative Medicine
     Monash University

     ALLEN CHENG
     Professor, Infectious Disease Epidemiology
     Monash University

2:20 p.m. **Q&A**

2:35 p.m.   **Understanding Legal and Regulatory Considerations of Border Mitigation**
STEVEN SOLOMON
Principal Legal Officer
World Health Organization

STEVEN HOFFMAN
Director
Global Strategy Lab
WHO Collaborating Centre on Global Governance of Antimicrobial Resistance;
Dahdaleh Distinguished Chair in Global Governance & Legal
Epidemiology

MATHIEU POIRIER
Associate Director
Global Strategy Lab

2:55 p.m.   **Q&A**

3:10 p.m.   **Perspectives from the Airline Industry**
TBD

3:25 p.m.   **Q&A**

3:35 p.m.   **Perspectives from the Cruise Industry**
RICHARD FAIN
CEO
Royal Caribbean Cruise Line
3:50 p.m. **Q&A**
4:00 p.m. **Perspectives from the Cruise Industry**

DONALD BROWN
VP, Maritime Policy
Cruise Lines International Association

4:15 p.m.   **Q&A**

4:25 p.m.   **Perspectives from the Cruise Industry**
FRANK DEL RIO
CEO
Norwegian Cruise Line

4:40 p.m.	**Q&A**
5:00 p.m.	**Adjourn**

Friday, January 21, 2022

OPEN SESSION

SESSION V—LEGAL CONSIDERATIONS

11:00 a.m.	**Welcome and Introduction from the Committee Chair** GEORGES C. BENJAMIN, *Committee Chair* Executive Director American Public Health Association
11:05 a.m.	**Legal Considerations** WILLIAM CHANG
11:20 a.m.	**Q&A**
11:45 a.m.	**Legal Considerations** GLENN COHEN Deputy Dean and James A. Attwood & Leslie Williams Professor of Law Harvard Law School
12:00 p.m.	**Q&A**
12:15 p.m.	**Center for Forecasting & Outbreak Analytics: Data & Evaluation** CAITLIN RIVERS ASSOCIATE DIRECTOR Center for Forecasting and Outbreak Analytics U.S. Centers for Disease Control and Prevention MARC LIPSITCH Executive Director Center for Forecasting and Outbreak Analytics U.S. Centers for Disease Control and Prevention
12:30 p.m.	**Q&A**
12:45 p.m.	**Break**

End of Open Session

February Meetings

February 10 and 11, 2022
February 10, 2022, 10 a.m. to 12 p.m. and 2 p.m. to 4 p.m. ET
February 11, 2022, 10 a.m. to 12 p.m. and 2 p.m. to 4 p.m. ET

Meeting Objectives

- Learn about DGMQ budget and workforce needs
- Hear perspectives from state and local DGMQ partners
- Review draft recommendations and identify research needs

Thursday, February 10, 2022—Meeting 4, Session 1

OPEN SESSION

SESSION I—PERSPECTIVES FROM STATE AND LOCAL PARTNERS

10:00 a.m.	**Welcome, Meeting's Objectives and Introduction** GEORGES C. BENJAMIN, *Committee Chair* Executive Director American Public Health Association
10:05 a.m.	**State and Local Partner Perspectives** MEREDITH ALLEN Vice President, Health Security Association of State and Territorial Health Officials
10:20 a.m.	LORI TREMMEL FREEMAN Chief Executive Director National Association of County and City Health Officials
10:35 a.m.	**Discussion with Committee** **End of Open Session**

APPENDIX B

Friday, February 11, 2022—Meeting 4, Session 2

OPEN SESSION

SESSION II—DGMQ FINANCE AND WORKFORCE OVERVIEW

10:00 a.m. **Welcome and Meeting's Objective**
GEORGES C. BENJAMIN, *Committee Chair*
Executive Director
American Public Health Association

10:05 a.m. **Overview of DGMQ Budget and Workforce Needs**
MARTIN CETRON
Director
Division of Global Migration and Quarantine
U.S. Centers for Disease Control and Prevention

BRIAN MASKERY
Health Economist
Division of Global Migration and Quarantine
U.S. Centers for Disease Control and Prevention

FRANCISCO ALVARADO-RAMY
Chief Medical Officer, Quarantine and Border Health Services
Division of Global Migration and Quarantine
U.S. Centers for Disease Control and Prevention

SHAHROKH ROOHI
Senior Advisor for Preparedness and Response
Division of Global Migration and Quarantine
Centers for Disease Control and Prevention

KARA TARDIVEL
Captain, United States Public Health Service
Maritime Unit Co-Lead, Global Migration Task Force
Acting Maritime Activity Lead, Quarantine and Border Health Services
Branch, Division of Global Migration and Quarantine
Centers for Disease Control and Prevention

JESSICA L. DAMON
CDR, U.S.PHS Commissioned Corps
Principal Management Officer
Division of Global Migration and Quarantine, Office of the Director

11:00 a.m.   **Discussion with Committee**

12:00 p.m.   **Break**

End of Open Session